Multiple
Sclerosis

Multiple Sclerosis

EVERYTHING YOU NEED TO KNOW

REVISED EDITION

PAUL O'CONNOR, MD, MSc, FRCPC

FIREFLY BOOKS

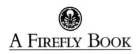

A FIREFLY BOOK

Published by Firefly Books (U.S.) Inc. 2005

First printing

Publisher Cataloging-in-Publication Data (U.S.)

Multiple sclerosis : everything you need to know / Paul O'Connor. –Rev. ed.
[168] p. : cm. (Your personal health)
Includes index.
Summary: Practical health guide to multiple sclerosis for both patients and their families, including advice on diagnosis, treatment options and symptoms.
ISBN 1-55297-889-3 (pbk.)
1. Multiple sclerosis -- Popular works. 2. Multiple sclerosis -- Treatment.
3. Multiple sclerosis -- Handbooks, manuals, etc. I. Title. II. Series.
616.834 dc22 RC377.O23 2005

Published in the United States by
Firefly Books (U.S.) Inc.
P.O. Box 1338, Ellicott Station
Buffalo, New York 14205

Published in Canada in 2005 by Key Porter Books Limited

Diagrams: Lianne Friesen
Electronic formatting: Heidy Lawrence Associates

Printed in Canada

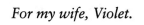

For my wife, Violet.

Contents

Acknowledgments / ix

Introduction / x

Chapter One: What Is MS? / 1

Chapter Two: What Causes MS? / 8

Chapter Three: How Does MS Affect You? / 17

Chapter Four: How Is MS Diagnosed? / 29

Chapter Five: Managing MS Symptoms / 40

Chapter Six: Treating the Disease:
               Present and Future / 102

Chapter Seven: Social Aspects of MS / 116

Chapter Eight: A Final Word / 132

Table of Drug Names / 135

Glossary / 137

Further Resources / 140

Index / 145

Acknowledgments

I would like to thank Gemma Asingua for her help in typing the manuscript. The staff of the Multiple Sclerosis Society of Canada read over the manuscript and provided many helpful suggestions.

Dr. R. Schapiro's invaluable book *Symptom Management in Multiple Sclerosis* was particularly helpful in the preparation of the chapter "Managing MS Symptoms" in this book.

Introduction

Typically, in modern medicine, we know a fair bit about who suffers from a condition, less about how to treat it effectively and least of all about what actually causes it. Certainly this applies to multiple sclerosis (MS), a disease of the nervous system that is the most common disabling neurological disorder of people between the ages of 20 and 40.

Jane is a 24-year-old store clerk. One day she notices poor vision in her right eye. It lasts for about six weeks and then clears. A year later she notes a numbness in her left arm and left leg. She also feels fatigued. She sees her family physician, who refers her to a neurologist. After diagnostic testing he tells her she has MS.

Bob is a 32-year-old stockbroker. He used to enjoy jogging, but in the past few years he has noticed a progressive stiffness and weakening in his legs which does not improve. He has also had urinary problems and sexual difficulties. He too sees a neurologist and, after a series of tests, learns that he has multiple sclerosis.

The Discovery of MS

The first description of what was probably MS dates back to August 4, 1421, when Jan Van Bieren, Count of Holland, described the "strange disease of the virgin Lidwina," who in

1395, at the age of 15, developed severe facial pain and leg weakness after falling on the ice while skating. Within a few years her problems had increased: her legs were so weak that she could not walk, she had leg numbness and she was intermittently blind in one eye. She died in 1433 at the age of 53.

The first descriptions of the physical changes that MS produces in the brain and spinal cord came almost simultaneously, in 1835, from Jean Cruveilhier, professor of pathologic anatomy in the Sorbonne's Faculty of Medicine in Paris, and Robert Carswell, a Scotsman who worked at the Hôpital de la Pitié in Paris for three years.

However, the first scientific description of the signs and symptoms of MS came from Jean-Martin Charcot (1825–1893). Charcot outlined a condition called *la sclérose en plaques*—in effect, multiple sclerosis—which he had first become familiar with while watching its gradual development in a maid employed in his house. From 1862 to 1870, Charcot worked at La Salpêtrière, a Paris asylum for beggars, the aged, the infirm and the insane. There, he examined thousands of patients. His findings led him to correlate the signs and symptoms of MS with the disease-related anatomical changes seen at autopsy.

Following Charcot's description, the disease was increasingly recognized. When the German pathologist Muller wrote a book on the subject in 1904, he cited more than 1,100 published papers relating to the subject.

Charcot's scientific exploration of MS paralleled the creation of neurology, the specialty branch of medicine that deals with diseases of the nervous system. In those early days, the only way to determine what was going on in a person was through neurological examination—that is, by having the person demonstrate how well certain functions of the nervous system (vision, balance, reflexes and so on) were working. Today we have a variety of special tests to help us diagnose the disease.

Types of MS

Charcot understood that MS is a variable disease with different forms. Today, physicians categorize MS as one of two main types. If recurrent attacks of neurological symptoms are followed by periods of improvement the disease is called *relapsing-remitting MS*. This is what Jane has. If, on the other hand, the symptoms worsen over time without any periods of improvement, the disease is called *progressive MS*. This is what Bob has. The types of MS will be explained in more detail in later chapters.

O N E

What Is MS?

What is happening in the nervous system of someone who has MS? Where is the damage done? Keeping in mind that we still don't know enough about the disease, here are the answers, based on our current level of knowledge.

The Nervous System

It would be impossible to overstate the importance to us of a normally functioning nervous system. This system is responsible for everything that makes us thinking, feeling, mobile beings. Different parts of the nervous system control different functions, so damage to particular areas results in loss of particular functions. To give a simple example: if the nervous tissue in your right eye is destroyed, you lose vision in your right eye.

The brain and spinal cord make up the *central nervous system* (CNS). From the CNS, nerves extend throughout the body to make up the *peripheral nervous system*. Significantly,

MS affects only the central nervous system. Comments in this book apply only to the central nervous system, unless otherwise noted.

The brain

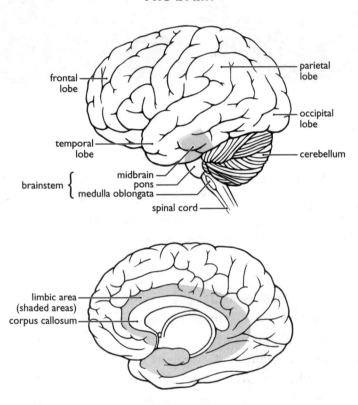

The brain itself consists of two main areas: a pair of hemispheres, on top, and the *brainstem*, on the bottom. The hemispheres (one on each side) are connected together by a bundle of fibers called the *corpus callosum*. Each hemisphere is divided into four main lobes, each of which has specialized functions. The *frontal lobes* are used mainly for planning, judgment and movement; the *temporal lobes* for memory; the *parietal lobes* for sensing; the *occipital lobes* for vision. Deep within the hemispheres lies the *limbic system*, an area involved in our emotions.

The brainstem carries electrical impulses from the hemispheres down to the nerves in the spinal cord, and from the spinal-cord nerves up to the hemispheres. Just behind the brainstem lies the *cerebellum*, the organ that controls our sense of balance and coordination.

How the Nervous System Works

The nervous system consists of billions of nerve cells called *neurons*, located mainly in the brain's *gray matter*. The gray matter covers the surface of the brain like the skin of an orange. The neurons communicate by sending electrical messages. These messages travel along a part of the neuron called the *axon*. Axons are located in the brain's *white matter*. The neuron connects with other neurons by sending messages across a gap called a *synapse*.

Nerve messages travel along axons the way telephone signals travel along a phone wire. This messaging process is repeated in billions of locations in each person's nervous system, all day, every day. Think of billions of interconnected electrical wires creating a system of linkages of unimaginable complexity. The human nervous system is exactly that.

Crucial in transmitting messages along the axons is a fatty protein called *myelin*. Just as phone wires require insulation so that the messages they convey do not dissipate, so too do axons. Myelin is the insulation of axons. This protein gets damaged in MS, and the damage is known as *demyelination*, which is why MS is called a demyelinating disease. Not only is the myelin damaged, resulting in a loss of electrical insulation. Even worse, the axon itself may be destroyed. Messages either get through slowly or do not get through at all.

Nerve cell

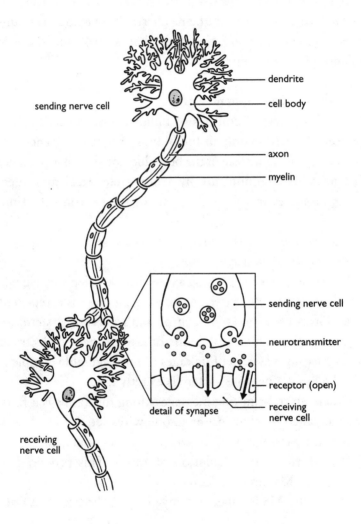

sending nerve cell

dendrite
cell body
axon
myelin

sending nerve cell
neurotransmitter
receptor (open)
receiving nerve cell

detail of synapse

receiving nerve cell

The symptoms of MS are caused by a combination of demyelination (losing the "insulation") and destruction of the axons (cutting the "wires" themselves). Much of the long-term, irreversible disability in MS comes from damage to the axons. Just as it's much easier to reinsulate a wire than to replace one that's been destroyed, it's a lot easier to remyelinate an axon than to get it to grow back and hook up with the right connections.

The Immune System

Why do the myelin and the axon get damaged in MS? To understand this, we have to know a bit about the *immune system*, an exceedingly complex, sophisticated and essential component that protects the human body from disease.

The immune system works on the premise that there are "self" tissues—which are "of the body"—and "nonself" tissues—which are not. The immune system does not tolerate "nonself" or foreign tissues, and relentlessly tries to destroy them. It is like an army that stands constantly on guard, continuously involved in skirmishes and ready for all-out war if necessary. The infantry in this army are the *lymphocytes*; the tanks are the *macrophages*. *B lymphocytes* use specialized proteins known as *antibodies* to destroy foreigners. *T lymphocytes* and *macrophages* prefer to engulf their enemies and destroy them chemically.

The infantry are roused to action when "scout" T lymphocytes encounter anything they deem to be foreign. Together with the macrophages, they produce molecules called *cytokines* that constantly signal the immunological army to either increase or decrease its activity at any given location, including the nervous system.

MS Is Probably an Autoimmune Disease

In MS, the immune system attacks the body's own myelin. It strips this insulating protein from the axon and often destroys the axon itself. However, the immune system does not attack all the brain and spinal-cord myelin at once. For reasons unknown, it attacks the myelin sporadically. The location and intensity of the attack are unpredictable, and vary greatly not only within a person but from one person to the next. In general, a person's symptoms mirror the extent of the myelin damage. These immunological attacks go on for decades— probably for the remainder of the person's life.

Why does the immune system attack the myelin? Unfortunately, we don't know. We do know, however, that every so often the immune system—despite its great complexity and elegance, or perhaps because of it—makes a mistake and starts a war against the body's own tissues. These "wars by mistake," called *autoimmune diseases*, include disorders of the joints (rheumatoid arthritis), thyroid gland (thyroiditis), stomach (pernicious anemia), pancreas (diabetes mellitus) and brain (multiple sclerosis). It may be that the immune system meets up with a foreign protein that closely resembles one of the body's myelin proteins, and then mistakenly attacks the myelin because it resembles that enemy protein. Viruses are thought to trigger autoimmune diseases, including MS, in this way. Or it may be that certain rogue elements in the immunological army become dysfunctional as a result of genetic mutations; they may stop "following orders," and embark on a misdirected campaign against the myelin.

It's not clear whether the immune system's attack on the myelin and the axons is the first step in this illness, or whether it follows some other problem in the nervous system. It could be that, for some reason, the myelin and the axons (or both) are already flawed in some subtle way, and that this flaw leads to the immune system's attack. Perhaps the myelin is somehow malformed so that it tends to fall apart, attracting the attention of the immune system. When we understand the exact cause of the disease, we will have more hope of finding effective treatments.

Steps in Demyelination

Destruction of the myelin, or demyelination, occurs in three steps:

1. the T lymphocytes migrate into (invade) the nervous system;
2. the T lymphocytes attack the myelin, with the help of macrophages;
3. the T lymphocytes produce cytokines to signal the rest of the army to become involved, resulting in a concentrated immune-system attack that causes inflammation and the formation of plaques, or permanent scars.

Why do we call this condition multiple sclerosis? "Multiple" signifies the many areas of inflammation and demyelination in the nervous system, and the repeated attacks of neurological symptoms over time. "Sclerosis" means scarring, and refers to the appearance of the brain and spinal cord when the disease has been present for some time, and repeated inflammation has left permanent scars.

What, then, is MS? Simply put, it is an autoimmune disease of the nervous system in which there is damage to both the myelin and the axons. Some of the axon damage is caused by the attacking immune system, and some is caused by degeneration, a premature "wearing out" process that results in axonal destruction.

T W O

What Causes MS?

Despite extensive research, we still don't know enough about what causes MS. However, we do know what factors are associated with the condition or seem to contribute to an increased risk of developing it. As with most medical conditions, they are both genetic (hereditary) and environmental. A genetically susceptible person encounters an environmental trigger and develops the disease.

Of course, just because one thing is *associated* with another, we cannot necessarily say that it *causes* the other. Living in North America, for instance, is associated with wearing a coat in winter (in most places, anyway). However, living in North America does not cause us to wear coats—the cold winter weather does. If for some reason the weather became much warmer, living in North America would no longer be associated with wearing a coat in winter. In looking at the possible causes of MS, we are examining associations that may or may not play a role in causing the condition.

Genetic Associations

Sex

Wherever multiple sclerosis occurs in the world, it is primarily a disease of young women. It is almost twice as common in women as it is in men. This is probably genetically determined, but why this is so remains unclear. Autoimmune diseases in general are more common in women.

Racial Group

Although MS occurs in all main racial groups, it is much more frequent in white people. It occurs most often in Caucasians in northern Europe and in those countries with Caucasians of northern European descent—Canada, the United States, Australia and New Zealand. However, MS is relatively uncommon in Caucasians in South Africa, northern areas of Australia and the southern United States. This suggests that racial group alone is not the sole factor in developing the disease.

In contrast, MS is uncommon in Asians and in blacks of African origin, though this is not to say that the condition never occurs. MS is also uncommon in Inuit, American Indians and Laplanders, even though they have lived for thousands of years in high-risk areas. This suggests that they are genetically protected from MS in some way.

Family History

In North America and northern Europe, about one person in a thousand has MS. This means that the baseline risk of getting MS if you live there is one in a thousand, or 0.1 percent. However, if you come from an ethnic group where MS is uncommon, your baseline risk is lower. On the other hand, if someone in your family has had MS, your risk increases.

The magnitude of the increase varies according to how close the affected relative is to you. If your sister or mother has MS, your risk of getting the disease is about 3 percent. Suppose your sister is actually a half-sister. This halves the risk to about 1.5 percent. What if you are adopted and your sister has MS? Then your risk falls right back to one in a thousand, or 0.1 percent. (These figures are an overall average; the risk is higher for female relatives than for male relatives.)

Now take the case of twins. Suppose your fraternal twin has MS. Because you are not genetically identical, your risk of getting MS is the same as that between siblings—3 percent. However, if your identical twin develops the condition, your risk of MS will be 30 percent. The more similar your genes are to those of a family member who has MS, the higher your risk.

A young woman diagnosed with MS is frequently concerned about passing on the condition to her children. The risk of her offspring developing MS is somewhere between 2 and 4 percent per child. Daughters have a slightly higher risk of developing

Is there an MS gene?

Using sophisticated technology, geneticists are now able to analyze the genome—the complete set of genes in a human being. This automated analysis allows them to look at the DNA from hundreds, if not thousands, of people. By analyzing families in which more than one person has MS, geneticists in Canada, the United States and Europe have found genes on two or more chromosomes that appear to make a person more likely to get MS. Unfortunately, there is no single "MS gene"—several, perhaps many genes are involved—so the genetic components of the disease are likely to remain difficult to sort out for many years, despite rapid advances in knowledge in this area.

the disease than sons have. Interestingly, the children of men with MS have, for reasons not yet explained, a lower risk of developing MS than the children of women with the disease.

Environmental Associations

Although genes play a role in getting MS, something else clearly triggers its development: namely, environmental factors. But while our genes are fixed, we can alter many environmental factors. This—at least in theory—may help us prevent the disease.

Latitude

Wherever MS is common in the world, one environmental factor is consistently present: a cool climate with relatively little sunshine. As latitude increases, multiple sclerosis becomes more common, with the highest incidence in areas above 40 degrees north latitude (around Denver or Philadelphia) and below 40 degrees south latitude. MS is more common in Canada and the northern U.S. than it is in the southern U.S.; more common in northern Europe than in southern Europe; more common in northern Japan than in southern Japan; and more common in southern Australia than in northern Australia (southern Australia is cooler than northern Australia because Australia is in the Southern Hemisphere).

Why is MS more common in cool latitudes? Researchers have tried repeatedly to identify which aspect of climate most strongly poses an increased risk for MS: temperature, sunshine, precipitation, humidity, altitude. When you consider these variables separately, each appears to affect the chance of multiple sclerosis. No one variable seems to dominate the picture, and because each affects the others, we can't really say which is most important.

Diet and MS

We know that people in cooler countries tend to be more affluent, and to have diets high in fat. A high-fat diet has been blamed for causing MS. But be wary of blaming a disease on diet; it's too easy, and it can leave those who are ill feeling guilty for their disease.

No systematic study has ever proved that a high-fat or high-dairy diet causes MS. If we compare countries as a whole we do find an association between the two. However, if we look *within* a country, this association vanishes. In fact, studies of the diets of people with MS prior to their developing the disease have in general shown that they are no different from the diets of other members of the population. Most Americans and Canadians who go to their doctor with their first episode of MS seem to eat a typically North American diet. Most are not vegetarians and most consume a moderate amount of meat and dairy products.

People with MS come in all sizes and weights, again suggesting that no one diet predisposes someone to the disease. But while diet has not been proved to cause MS, it has not been ruled out as a modifying factor. For example, it's possible that exposure to certain foods early in life may, in some individuals, trigger MS later. Perhaps because the food we eat is such a highly modifiable environmental factor, research on diet as a risk factor continues. The question of diet as a cause (or treatment) remains unresolved, and deserves further study.

Recently, there has been much interest in hours of sunshine per year, and in lack of sunshine as perhaps *the* environmental trigger in a genetically susceptible person. This factor seems to fit the data best, and sunshine is known to affect both the immune system and the body's synthesis of vitamin D—a nutrient that may play a role in protecting against MS.

It does seem likely that the link between multiple sclerosis and latitude is an indirect one. Latitude influences hours of sunshine, diet, housing design, means of sanitation, social customs and many other aspects of life. One or more of these factors, acting on a susceptible individual, may be the true connection between climate and MS. We do know that, whatever environmental factor(s) may trigger MS, it acts on a population level—that is, everyone in the population is exposed to the factor, whatever it may be.

Socioeconomic Status

MS tends to occur more commonly in people in middle to upper socioeconomic brackets. This is an association, rather than a cause, and we don't know what the connection is. MS also seems to be more common among city dwellers than among rural folk. Again, nobody knows why.

Infections

As explained earlier, it may be that the immune system mistakes myelin for a virus, and attacks it, so that the virus causes MS indirectly. But some physicians believe that viruses cause MS directly. They believe that MS is a delayed reaction to a viral infection contracted during childhood by a genetically susceptible person. Over the years, researchers have suggested that different viruses, including measles, chicken pox, shingles and certain other herpes viruses, might be involved. A more subtle and intriguing version of the viral theory suggests that it is not so much having the viral infection that triggers MS but the *age* at which you get it. Thus, if you have a viral infec-

---

Allergies and MS are probably not linked

There is no convincing statistical evidence that people with MS are any more "allergic" than other members of the population. Some have one or two allergies, many have none and a few have many allergies—just like the population as a whole. Whether MS represents an allergic response to certain dietary proteins—a popular and appealingly simple idea— remains to be established.

tion such as measles or chicken pox when you're young, the risk of developing MS is low. On the other hand, if you're older, your risk of developing MS is higher. This theory fits interestingly with the geographic distribution of MS. In general, children living in warm countries are, for a variety of reasons, exposed to common viruses at a younger age than are children in cool countries. Perhaps their early exposure protects them against MS.

We do know that the severity of an infection frequently varies according to the age at which you get the infection. For example, infection with the polio virus early in life commonly causes no significant disease; infection later in childhood substantially increases the risk of complications such as paralysis.

A connection between multiple sclerosis and the age of infected children would also explain the socioeconomic data. Because standards of sanitation are higher and the amount of

Mystery in the Faeroes

Occasionally, there is an outbreak of MS in a small community. The most famous one occurred in the Faeroes, a group of islands lying between Norway and Iceland. No MS had ever been reported there until 1943, at which point several cases appeared. Between 1940 and 1945, British troops occupied the Faeroes. It turned out that most of the Faeroese who developed MS lived close to where the troops were stationed. Was there something about the British occupation that triggered MS in this previously unaffected population? No one really knows, but the outbreak raised the possibility that one group (the British) transmitted an agent to another (the Faeroese) that caused the MS. Epidemiologists have greatly debated the subject over the years. They don't know which environmental factor, if any, is the culprit. The main suspect was an infectious agent, such as a virus, that seemed to cause problems only in younger people. Generally, though, MS is not transmitted between spouses, family or friends. If a virus is involved, it's at work early in life.

living space is greater in the chillier developed world, common childhood infections tend to occur later in life there, particularly in middle-income and upper-income groups. The problem with the viral theory is that, despite a huge amount of work, no one has ever provided convincing evidence that a virus, or any other infectious agent, actually causes MS.

Migration

Information from people who have moved from countries where MS is uncommon, such as Jamaica, to countries where MS is common, such as England, enables us to look at MS susceptibility from another point of view. Until recently, researchers believed that the age at which you moved was pivotal to your risk of MS. If you moved before the age of 15, your risk seemed to be that of people in the country you moved to. If you moved after the age of 15, your risk seemed fixed at that of the country you grew up in. Now the connection has become a little less clear. It may be more correct to say that, geographically, your risk of MS is more a function of where you are now, than where you grew up.

Research into the cause of MS continues, and scientists are optimistic that they will find an answer to at least part of the puzzle in the near future. Why are they having such difficulty making progress? It may be that the biological process by which MS develops is unique to this disease; perhaps we haven't discovered it because we don't know exactly where to look, or how. My own hunch, for what it's worth, is that genetic factors will be increasingly recognized as important in this disease. I also believe that the environmental trigger is directly related to how sunny the climate is where you live or lived in the past. The amount of sunshine affects how much Vitamin D is in your body, which may be important in triggering MS, although this has not been completely proven. Everyone is exposed to the environmental factor that causes MS, but genetic predisposition—or even gene changes (mutations)—may determine who develops the disease, and how severe it becomes. Whatever the cause may be, we are certainly making progress in diagnosing MS and treating its symptoms. We are even—finally—learning to treat the disease itself.

THREE

How Does MS Affect You?

U nlike many other diseases, MS causes a multitude of signs and symptoms. This is because this inflammatory disease attacks the myelin of the central nervous system (brain, brainstem and spinal cord). The CNS is exquisitely specialized, with different parts responsible for different functions, so the signs and symptoms vary depending on the specific areas of the CNS being affected. For example, if an attack happens to hit the eye (optic) nerve, vision may be lost in that eye. This diversity is one of the reasons MS is hard to diagnose.

Although there is no such thing as a typical case of MS, it is possible to give a general account of how the condition evolves. In 90 percent of all cases, symptoms begin between the ages of 20 and 40. The first symptom is often loss of vision in one eye for a few weeks, or numbness of the limbs for that time. It comes on insidiously and you may not even recognize it as being significant. Frequently, people don't seek medical attention—or if they do, the problem has often resolved itself

Symptoms and signs: what's the difference?

Strictly speaking, *symptoms* are feelings you yourself notice, such as pain, weakness or loss of sensation. They are subjective—different people experience and report them differently—and prone to misinterpretation by you or your physician. *Signs* are specific abnormalities your physician detects when he or she examines you. They are objective, and serve as useful markers of the presence of disease. In many instances, signs independently explain or confirm the significance of symptoms. The search for signs is the reason a neurologist examines your eyes and tests your strength, sensation, reflexes and balance.

by the time the examination occurs, so that the physician finds nothing wrong. Recovery seems complete after this first attack, which is called a *clinically isolated syndrome* (CIS).

Weeks or even decades may pass before a second attack. Further attacks follow. With each successive attack, recovery tends to be incomplete. Finally, you seek medical attention again and your family physician refers you to a neurologist. Further diagnostic evaluation confirms the presence of MS. This is called *relapsing-remitting* MS.

After another variable period of time—perhaps 10 to 20 years or more—you may enter the *secondary progressive* phase of the illness. This is characterized by a slow increase in disability without remissions (periods of recovery). Fortunately, about 20 percent of relapsing-remitting patients never enter the progressive phase of the disease. The average person with MS has one attack of symptoms every year or two, although this varies widely among individuals. The greatest number of attacks comes during the first few years after diagnosis, and then the number of attacks settles down. Although the disease seems to lurch between attack and recovery, tests using diagnostic imaging (see Chapter Four) indicate that

Common symptoms of MS

- fatigue
- depression
- memory changes
- pain
- visual loss
- double vision
- unsteadiness and dizziness
- weakness
- shaking and loss of coordination
- numbness and tingling
- bladder problems
- bowel problems
- sexual problems

attacks of inflammation in the nervous system are more or less continuous, even in the absence of clinical symptoms. However, the rate at which new areas of inflammation develop varies, both for one individual, and from person to person. Each attack of inflammation causes damage to an area of myelin and axons.

The description above is true for about 85 percent of all cases; the MS begins with attacks of symptoms that improve spontaneously with time. In the other 15 percent of cases, the symptoms come on slowly but do not improve. This pattern is called *primary progressive* because the disease is progressive right from the start, instead of being secondary to a relapsing-remitting phase.

Here, in greater detail, are the symptoms of MS.

Fatigue

Barbara is a 32-year-old woman with MS. She feels "tired all the time." She isn't just tired at the end of the day or after going for a long walk. After working for as little as two hours, she feels mentally and physically drained and has to take a break. The fatigue is slowly worsening. If she catches a cold or has some other illness, she feels a lot more worn out than other people do. At the end of the day she is exhausted, and she is usually in bed by nine o'clock.

Fatigue is probably the most common symptom in MS. It is often described as an overwhelming worn-out feeling or a generalized weakness. Most important, it usually comes on after only one or two hours of being up. Just getting washed and having breakfast are enough to make many people feel they need a break. The fatigue is relieved partially by rest. People often sleep extra hours at night, and they may have a nap or two in the daytime.

The exact cause of the fatigue in MS has never been identified. It may be due to a number of factors: the disease itself, reduced muscle strength or endurance, and depression. It may be worse in warm, humid weather. It can be quite disabling and definitely interferes with productivity at work or at home. This in turn may lead to feelings of guilt or depression. Fatigue contributes significantly to the disability of MS. Because they are vague, subjective and hard to measure, the debilitating effects of fatigue do not receive the respect from others, including insurance companies, that they deserve.

Depression

After developing a loss of vision in her right eye and weakness in her legs—early symptoms of MS—Catherine becomes significantly depressed. Her appetite decreases and her sleep is not restful, even though she feels tired all the time. She becomes completely uninterested in sex with her husband. Feelings of guilt and worthlessness follow, to the point where she contemplates suicide. Then her doctor puts her on antidepressants, and within a few weeks her mood brightens. She is able to enjoy her family and friends again.

All of us feel sad or blue from time to time. When physicians refer to depression, they mean a more severe kind of sadness or downbeat mood. It is often associated with other symptoms such as a disturbance in appetite, energy level, sleep or sexual desire. Sometimes it is masked by an outward appearance of cheerfulness, even excessive cheerfulness.

Depression is common in MS, and probably affects half of those with the disease at some point in their illness. At any given moment, about 12 percent of those with MS are seriously depressed, compared with 5 percent of the general population. Suicide is three to ten times more common in people with MS. This is especially tragic as MS usually strikes those who are young and have many years of life left. People with more severe disabilities are, quite naturally, more prone to depression. Fortunately, this type of depression often responds well to treatment.

Memory Changes

Joe is a high-school math teacher who prides himself on his ability to remember his work schedule without having to make notes. When he develops MS, he begins to have more and more difficulty doing this. Several times he forgets important engagements, which of course angers his employer. He has trouble concentrating on a task for more than a short while, and has slightly more difficulty explaining concepts to his students.

MS is a disease of the brain, so it's not surprising that it is associated with symptoms of cognitive dysfunction such as decreased memory, attention and concentration, and difficulty putting thoughts into words. The degree of cognitive dysfunction reflects the extent of the disease in the brain, particularly in the frontal and temporal lobes. MS affects white-matter connections in these lobes and produces short circuits that show up as difficulties with cognition. Still, many people have absolutely no problems with memory or other cognitive functions despite significant MS.

Pain

Elizabeth has had MS for five years. One day she wakes up with a burning pain in both legs. It is not severe but it certainly is irritating. She finds it difficult to wear panty hose because they worsen the burning. The pain is constantly present, although it varies in degree. Fred, on the other hand, has a jabbing pain in parts of his face. Although the pain lasts only a few seconds at a time, it is excruciating and causes him to seek help. Medication soon brings the pain under control.

People with MS frequently complain of pain. Distinguishing the pain of MS from other pain is difficult. Pain that is sharp, burning and localized—affecting, for example, one limb or another—may be due to MS. However, pain from other causes—a slipped disc, for instance—may resemble the pain of MS, and such factors need to be ruled out. Pain that occurs with numbness and tingling is much more likely to be due to a neurological problem such as MS than to strained muscles or arthritic joints. Aching pain is not directly due to MS, but may occur because of muscle and joint stiffness related to the disease.

Visual Loss

Gina is 18 years old, a happy and healthy university student. One day she notices that her vision in one eye seems slightly "washed out." She describes this as "a film over my eye." She also notices pain in that eye, particularly if she moves it from side to side. Over the next two days, the pain and visual loss worsen and she becomes alarmed. To her immense relief, her vision rapidly improves, and by the time she goes to her doctor it is back to normal, with the pain gone. Listening to her story, her physician is nonetheless concerned and sends her to a neurologist, who tells her that she had an inflammation of her optic nerve.

Visual loss due to MS occurs because the optic nerve, which connects the brain to the eye, becomes inflamed. Physicians call this *optic neuritis*. Typically, you lose sight in the center of the visual field. It usually happens in only one eye at a time, often with an aching pain in that eye. It may be experienced as a persistent fogginess of vision. However, visual loss due to MS is not at all the same as the temporary blurring you sometimes have with headaches or when your eyes are tired. Nor is it the same as the loss of sight, for a few minutes or longer, that occurs during migraines. Visual loss due to MS lasts from days to weeks, and visual loss lasting less than this is not usually due to optic neuritis.

Double Vision

Harold has never had much difficulty with his MS. However, about two weeks after having a cold, he notices that when he looks to the right he sees double. If he looks to the left there is no problem. Looking up and down are also okay, and he has no pain. He correctly suspects that the double vision is due to his MS, and his neurologist explains that he is having a relapse. With corticosteroid treatment (see Chapter Six) he soon regains his normal vision.

Sometimes people with MS suffer from double vision. The two images may exist side by side or one on top of the other. Like visual loss, double vision has to last for days to weeks before it is attributed to MS.

Unsteadiness and Dizziness

Isabel is a bicycle courier with mild MS. One day, as she stands up, the whole room seems to be spinning. Even when she stays absolutely still, the spinning continues. She feels nauseated, and vomits twice that day. When she walks, she is unsteady and tends to stagger. Her roommate tells her she looks "drunk." Isabel sees her neurologist, and with treatment she soon feels steady again.

Vertigo—a condition in which you feel you or your surroundings are whirling—afflicts some people with MS. It is often associated with a feeling of unsteadiness. Incoordination of arms, legs, walking and speech can occur even without dizziness, and is a major cause of disability (see below).

Weakness

Mary is a 38-year-old nurse. One morning she notices a slight weakness in her right leg. Over the next two or three days this evolves into complete paralysis of that leg. A year ago she had an episode of blurred vision in her left eye that lasted for two or three weeks. After appropriate investigations, she is told that she has MS. The right leg problem clears partially over the next six weeks, although some weakness persists.

Multiple sclerosis may cause weakness of the arms, legs and/or face. This weakness may occur on one entire side of the body—for example, the right arm, right leg and right side of the face. It may involve just a single limb, such as the leg, or it may affect all four limbs. The degree of weakness is variable, ranging from complete paralysis to only a slight loss of strength. The weakness may come on slowly, over a period of years, or suddenly, in a matter of hours.

Shaking and Loss of Coordination

One day Kirsten, who has had MS for six years, notices that her right arm is shaking uncontrollably as she brings her soupspoon to her mouth. When she tries to walk she is unsteady, although her legs feel strong. She staggers and needs to use a cane. Soon, using a cane becomes permanently necessary, and although Kirsten continues to walk, she is very self-conscious about her ability and avoids walking on uneven surfaces or stairs. Since the shaking in her right hand started, she has had trouble with buttons, and her handwriting has worsened as well.

MS may cause incoordination of the arms and legs. Sometimes walking balance is affected. People with MS may find it impossible to ride a bicycle or go up and down stairs safely. Handwriting may deteriorate and fine motor activities such as doing up or undoing buttons or putting a key in a lock may be difficult. Sometimes speech becomes slurred. It may also be hard to swallow food.

Numbness and Tingling

Clare is a 25-year-old woman who developed numbness in her feet that spread upward to involve her legs, and her abdomen up to her belly button. The symptoms came on over three days. "It feels like I'm wearing a tight pair of panty hose," she said. She also had bowel and bladder problems. These symptoms all cleared over the next two weeks. The changes in sensation and bowel and bladder function were caused by inflammatory demyelination in her spinal cord, something her doctor called *myelitis*.

Joan, a 32-year-old librarian who had her first child eight months ago, has just begun to notice that, whenever she bends her head forward, she experiences a shock-like sensation down her spine and legs. She didn't notice this during her pregnancy or delivery, or even in those first few tiring months after the birth.

From time to time all of us experience numbness or tingling, often because of the way we are sitting or lying. We adjust our position and these symptoms disappear. Numbness or sensory changes associated with MS, on the other hand, may last for days to weeks. Joan's problem, called *Lhermitte's sign*—a tingling electric feeling in the spine, arms and sometimes the legs, caused by flexing the neck—is quite common in MS.

Bladder, Bowel and Sexual Problems

Lillian has MS. The main problems have been numbness of the legs and some temporary loss of vision, but now she has begun to notice that unless she is careful, she loses urine from her bladder. She also finds that instead of going to the bathroom three or four times a day, she has to go eight or nine times each day. This is troubling, and she finds herself needing to wear a pad at all times to avoid embarrassment. At first she thinks she has a urinary infection, but tests are negative. Her family doctor refers her to a urologist, who informs her, after testing, that her incontinence is due to the MS. With help she learns to manage her urinary problems.

Michael has MS that causes weakness and numbness in his legs. As if this were not enough to cope with, he has begun to notice a decline in his ability to perform sexually. He is frequently impotent, and as a result is worried and embarrassed. Even when he gets an erection, he sometimes wilts at the critical moment and is unable to ejaculate. Fortunately he has an understanding partner, who suggests that he seek treatment. He is provided with a number of treatment options, and his performance soon returns to a nearly normal level.

Bladder problems are common in MS. They include frequency (urinating as often as every 15 to 20 minutes, usually in small amounts); dribbling (leaking small amounts); urgency (not being

Special features of MS symptoms

- MS symptoms worsen with exposure to heat. For example, John experiences a loss of vision in his right eye that clears completely after six weeks. However, he notices that whenever he has a hot bath or gets particularly hot working out, the visual disturbance recurs and persists until he cools down. Leslie finds that although her legs are weak all the time, they are especially weak after she has a hot bath or a shower. In fact, she has difficulty walking for the first half-hour afterward. This worsening of symptoms when you are exposed to heat is called *Uhthoff's phenomenon* and is common. Why it happens is unclear, but the heat probably reduces nerve transmissions along axons that have lost their myelin.
- MS symptoms tend to worsen with fatigue. In general, people with MS feel much better in the morning. As the day wears on they become tired and their symptoms become worse. Fever, depression or just feeling stressed can all worsen symptoms significantly.
- MS symptoms tend to come on spontaneously, then disappear spontaneously. The onset of symptoms is called a *relapse*. Their disappearance is called a *remission*. Precisely why remission occurs is hotly debated. Recovery may be due to remyelination of demyelinated axons, or the axon may have repair mechanisms that allow it to transmit signals better even though there is demyelination. Or the swelling in the inflamed areas of the brain may go down, causing less pressure on the axon.

able to wait to void); hesitancy (being slow to start voiding); incontinence (spontaneous urination); urinary infection (painful burning during urination, with or without fever). There may also be bowel problems, such as constipation or diarrhea. Sexual problems are common too.

Brief Symptoms of MS

Almost all MS symptoms occur over days to weeks to months. Occasionally, however, people with MS develop unusual symptoms that last for only a few seconds to a few minutes: for example, lightning-like episodes of pain and tingling; intermittent slurring of speech; brief weakness and unsteadiness; even cramplike spasms of the arms and legs.

In about 5 percent of cases, people with MS develop seizures. These can take many different forms. Here is one example. Nellie has MS, but it has not caused her too much trouble. One day she develops significant weakness of her right arm and right leg, then shaking of the right arm and right leg. A full-blown convulsion follows. Her body becomes rigid and she temporarily turns blue. The convulsion lasts for only a minute or so, during which time she is unconscious, bites her tongue and empties her bladder. When she wakes up she feels tired and confused, and has no memory of what has just happened. Medication prevents further seizures.

An important warning here: having one, or even several, of the symptoms mentioned in this chapter does not mean you have MS. Some of the symptoms are so general that there isn't a person alive who hasn't had them at some time or other. All of us have felt tired, weak, numb, unsteady or dizzy from time to time, and only one of us in a thousand has MS. The disease can be diagnosed reliably only with a neurological examination and confirmatory testing.

F O U R

How Is MS Diagnosed?

Diagnosing MS will require the help of your family physician and usually a neurologist. They'll use a number of tests, but the most important information will come from your medical history and your neurological examination. Because MS occurs in a part of the body that is hard to access—the brain and spinal cord—any evidence of its presence is necessarily indirect. To complicate matters, different areas of the nervous system are affected in different people. It is often difficult to detect the disease with just one test. People frequently rely more on diagnostic tests than on the judgment of the physician, but the fact is that every MS diagnosis is a matter of judgment. Just as a judge in a court case must weigh every piece of evidence and come up with a verdict, so the physician—usually a neurologist—must weigh all the evidence and come up with a diagnosis. The difficulty of diagnosing MS explains why some people go for years having neurological symptoms but not knowing they have MS, and why one neurologist may tell them they have the disease while

What is a neurologist?

A neurologist is a physician who has five or more years of extra training, after medical school, in diseases of the nervous system. Neurologists are involved in the diagnosis and treatment of diseases of the brain, spinal cord and peripheral nervous system. They are often confused with neurosurgeons, but neurosurgeons perform operations on the nervous system, whereas neurologists use medical treatments such as medications or other therapies. Since multiple sclerosis is a disease restricted to the nervous system, and since most of the treatments do not involve surgery, neurologists are the specialists who manage this illness.

another may say they don't. Understandably, people find this uncertainty very frustrating.

The Diagnostic Process

MS frequently begins slowly. Symptoms may be present for months or years before they are brought to the attention of a physician. These early symptoms are often so mild or vague that even a physician doesn't recognize their significance, though sometimes they are more severe and their onset is more abrupt. At some point your family physician will refer you to a neurologist. The neurologist will first take a full history to review your current symptoms, your previous illnesses, your use of medication and any family history of neurological disease. Your social situation will also be considered, to identify any causes of stress or depression that might influence the symptoms. A neurological examination will follow, during which the neurologist evaluates eye and face movements, reflexes and limb strength, sensation and coordination, and determines what, if any, further testing is necessary. Remember the analogy of the judge deciding on a court case. Each piece of evidence must be weighed, and in the end the diagnosis is a matter of judgment.

Confirmatory Diagnostic Tests

Magnetic Resonance Imaging (MRI)

Nowadays, virtually anyone suspected of having MS undergoes imaging of the nervous system, usually with a procedure called *magnetic resonance imaging*. MRI is by far the most useful diagnostic test developed to date for this disease, for it reveals the structure of the nervous system in startling detail. Multiple sclerosis typically produces small areas of abnormality, particularly in regions of the brain and spinal cord rich in myelin. These lesions show up as dots on the scan and are readily apparent to a skilled neurologist. Because the magnetic resonance scanner uses a powerful magnet to generate this picture, if you have any metal in your head or body it may not be possible to perform the test. Sometimes a chemical called a *contrast agent* is injected to enhance the amount of information obtained. During the test you will lie for 15 to 30 minutes in a small enclosed area. People who are severely claustrophobic usually find they cannot complete the test. The test is also moderately noisy. Scanning is not generally done during pregnancy.

An MRI scan of the brain will usually show abnormalities if MS is present. Unfortunately, in up to 25 percent of early cases the disease does not show up. In addition, the pattern of abnormality on an MRI scan is not absolutely specific for MS; other conditions, even normal aging, sometimes mimic the changes of MS. Like any other test, the MRI is not perfect, and the neurologist will have to make a judgment call. MRIs of the spinal cord are also sometimes helpful in making a diagnosis.

Evoked Potentials

In *evoked potentials* tests, wires are attached to the scalp, neck and limbs, and visual, hearing and feeling pathways are stimulated. These tests record how quickly and completely the nerve signals provoked by the stimulation reach the brain. In MS, signal transmission usually slows down somewhat and the transmitted signal is weaker. The test shows abnormalities in the function of nerve pathways in about 65 percent of cases of early MS. It is especially useful when findings on the MRI scan are unexpectedly normal or borderline. The equipment for this testing is much less expensive than that for MRI and in general the test is simpler to do. No needles or injections are involved, and there is no radiation. The test takes one to two hours. The only discomfort is a slight tingling of the arms and legs during stimulation. It is safe to do even during pregnancy.

Spinal Fluid Examination

Sometimes the spinal fluid is examined to check for special proteins called *immunoglobulins*. These proteins are produced by B lymphocytes. Since the latter are overactive in the central nervous system of a person with MS, a high level of immunoglobulins in the spinal fluid is an indicator of the disease. To get the fluid, a long needle is inserted at the base of the spine and a few drops of fluid are drawn. The procedure is called a *spinal tap*.

Some people are understandably reluctant to undergo this test because it involves discomfort. In addition, people sometimes have headaches for a few days afterward. However, the information obtained can be extremely helpful in sorting out cases where the MRI and evoked potentials results are inconclusive.

Computerized Axial Tomography (CT) Scan

A *CT scan* is another way of taking a picture of the brain. It involves the use of radiation and is no longer employed as a test for MS. It is still sometimes used to rule out other brain abnormalities, where MRI is not readily available. The test lasts 15 to 30 minutes, and should not be performed during pregnancy.

There are no blood tests available that indicate whether MS is present, but blood tests may be performed to rule out other conditions that might mimic this disease. However, blood test results very rarely change a diagnosis of suspected MS into something else.

What Does a Diagnosis of MS Mean?

The phrase "multiple abnormalities in time and space" sums up what a physician needs to find to make a diagnosis of MS. In other words, you must exhibit neurological abnormalities in different parts of the nervous system on different occasions for MS to be diagnosed. For example, there might be loss of vision one month, caused by inflammation in the optic nerve, and vertigo three months later, caused by inflammation in the brainstem—each confirmed by a neurological exam and testing, as necessary. When you have such a pattern of symptoms and signs, and other conditions have been ruled out, you are said to have MS. The findings of an MRI scan, evoked potentials test and spinal tap can help show the presence of one or more abnormalities in the nervous system. MS can be diagnosed after just one attack if, over time, MRI scans show that new lesions have developed, even if those lesions haven't caused new attacks. If you have had only one neurological attack, you are said to have *possible* MS. The diagnosis changes from possible MS to MS when you have further attacks, or when MRI scans show more lesions developing.

Only some people with possible MS ever go on to develop full-blown MS. Given the huge impact of a diagnosis of MS,

Diagnosing MS

Under a recently developed set of rules called the *McDonald criteria*, a diagnosis of "MS," "possible MS" or "not MS" is based on MRI findings and the number of attacks, and the results of the evoked potentials and spinal fluid tests. In essence, the more abnormalities you have, the more likely you are to have MS, especially if the abnormalities develop over time.

both psychologically and socially, neurologists are reluctant to use this label prematurely. Telling people they have MS when in fact they do not leads to unnecessary stress and alarm. On the other hand, not telling people the possible cause of their symptoms is usually not helpful either. Every person's situation and desire for information are different, and the approach should be tailored to the individual. Nowadays, neurologists are very likely to tell patients as soon as possible that they may have MS, because early treatments may be helpful and because people have a right to know the state of their health. Previously, when there were no treatments anyway, the diagnosis was often delayed, in a perhaps misguided effort to spare the patient the worry that follows such unwelcome news.

In general, a diagnosis of MS causes several different reactions. Some people feel vindicated. This is the "I knew I wasn't crazy" reaction. Because of the stealthy way MS comes on, they have often been told by physicians that their symptoms are due to "bad nerves" or other psychological factors. Other people feel relieved that something even more sinister is not present. All the same, a diagnosis of MS conjures up frightening and very real concerns for the person involved and his or her family. Some people become anxious and depressed. Those whose MS is diagnosed at an early, mild stage, when it could well have been overlooked, sometimes talk about the diagnosis "ruining" their enjoyment of their lives. As with any serious diagnosis, most people have a mix of feelings that varies from hour to hour, day to day.

Conditions That May Be Confused with MS

A number of conditions resemble MS superficially, causing fatigue, weakness and/or numbness. Fatigue plays a major role in chronic fatigue syndrome, but MS and chronic fatigue syndrome are *not* the same thing; the latter does not cause abnormal results in a neurological examination, and MRI tests, as well as evoked potentials and spinal fluid, should be normal. Lyme disease is a bacterial infection that causes skin and joint abnormalities, but a neurological exam will implicate the peripheral nervous system, whereas MS affects the central nervous system. AIDS has nothing to do with MS; in fact, it is the opposite of MS in some respects. It involves an impaired immune system, rather than an overactive one. Someone with AIDS will test positive for HIV, and will not have spontaneous remissions of neurological symptoms.

Stroke results from a blocked or burst blood vessel and is completely unrelated to MS. Although stroke can cause abnormalities in MRI scans, they are different in appearance from those seen in MS. Also, stroke usually affects people who are considerably older. The abnormalities of lymphoma, a rare tumor of the lymph gland, likewise look different on MRI, and there is no spontaneous remission of lymphoma symptoms. A rare inflammatory condition called sarcoidosis can resemble MS in some respects, but it also shows up in other body systems, such as the lungs. The same is true of systemic lupus erythematosus, a chronic disease that affects the skin, blood vessels and joints.

Conditions that may be confused with MS

- chronic fatigue syndrome
- Lyme disease
- AIDS
- stroke
- psychological problems
- sarcoidosis
- systemic lupus erythematosus
- lymphoma

Sometimes psychological problems—particularly stress and/or depression—create symptoms that mimic MS, including fatigue, tingling, numbness and a generalized weakness, but again a neurological exam and an MRI and evoked potentials test will show no abnormalities. Part of the neurologist's job is distinguishing the similar symptoms of these conditions, and others, from the characteristics of multiple sclerosis.

What Will Happen to You If You Have MS?

People with MS naturally ask their physicians how the disease will affect them. However, it's impossible to give useful information about the long-term outlook immediately after the diagnosis, because MS varies from one person to the next and within one person over time.

After about five years, physicians have a much better idea of how the disease will evolve. Generally, the progress of the disease breaks down into the Rule of One-Third: One-third of people with MS do very well—their condition is sometimes called "benign MS"—one-third do moderately well and one-third are significantly disabled. Twenty years after diagnosis, about a sixth are in a wheelchair and half require some assistance with walking, be it cane, walker or wheelchair. Twenty-five years after diagnosis, two-thirds are still able to walk, although some need a cane or a walker and one-third use a wheelchair most of the time.

Clinical categories of multiple sclerosis

Clinically Isolated Syndrome (CIS)
There is a single attack of symptoms, but often multiple lesions are seen on the brain MRI. The earliest form of MS.

Relapsing-remitting MS (RRMS)
Attacks (relapses) of symptoms are followed by complete or partial improvement. There is no worsening between attacks.

A subtype of RRMS is *benign MS*, in which remission after relapses is almost complete, so that 10–15 years after the onset of the disease there is still only minimal disability. In most cases of benign MS, the symptoms mainly affect the senses of sight and/or touch. The proportion of MS patients who still have benign disease decreases with time, from 60 percent after 10 years, to 40 percent after 20 years, to 25 percent after 30 years.

Progressive MS
Disability slowly and continuously increases, with or without relapses.

In *primary progressive MS*, disability slowly increases right from the start of the disease. A rare subtype of primary progressive is *progressive-relapsing MS*, in which relapses occur during a course that is progressive from the onset of the disease. Primary progressive MS generally appears in people in their forties, and is the only form of MS that affects men and women equally.

In *secondary progressive MS*, the disease becomes progressive after an initial relapsing-remitting phase. Eventually (after 5–25 years or more) most people with relapsing-remitting MS develop secondary progressive MS. Confusingly, the term *relapsing-progressive* is used to describe secondary progressive MS in which sudden relapses occur during the course of gradual worsening. Relapsing-progressive is *not* the same as progressive relapsing.

Remember that MS comes in two main different forms: relapsing-remitting and progressive. Because treatment is determined by the kind of MS you have, it's important to ask your neurologist which of the four categories—clinically isolated, relapsing-remitting, primary progressive or secondary progressive—you are dealing with. At any given moment, about half of MS patients have relapsing-remitting MS and the other half have progressive MS. Relapsing-remitting disease can be highly variable. Progressive disease can be progressive right from the start (primary progressive) or can become progressive after being relapsing-remitting for many years. Progressive MS, of course, implies a progressive increase in disability. However, MS does not progress endlessly. After a variable length of time it usually plateaus, with no significant increase in disability. People with progressive MS are more likely to need a wheelchair and to have significant neurological disability. People who have remissions from their attacks usually have mild to moderate disability.

A number of other factors affect the prognosis. Perhaps most important are the specific symptoms you have. If they relate mainly to sensations such as feeling or vision, disability is usually moderate to mild. If the main symptoms are limb weakness and loss of coordination, you are more likely to become disabled eventually. Frequent attacks and failure to improve after attacks also suggest eventual disability.

In general, men with MS do worse than women with MS. No one knows why. Also, the later in life you come down with MS, the faster the neurological symptoms tend to get worse.

The most significant indicator of the prognosis is whether your condition is progressive, as a progressive course implies a greater degree of neurological disability. Progressive MS tends to develop at the same rate regardless of whether it is primary progressive or secondary progressive. These two are best thought of, not as different categorizations of MS, but simply as different stages.

To date, the MRI scan, evoked potentials test and spinal fluid examination can't predict the future with any accuracy. Refinements in our understanding of prognostic factors are allowing us to pick out some of the people who need more aggressive (and potentially risky) treatment, such as chemo-therapy or bone marrow transplantation.

Maybe the most important point about the prognosis in MS is that it is not as bad, on average, as most people think. We tend to notice the people who are most disabled by MS. Yet many people—co-workers, friends, relatives—live completely normal, full lives, with little or no visible disability.

FIVE

Managing MS Symptoms

I t is important to remember that not all your health problems are caused by MS. People with MS are as susceptible as others to colds, flus, broken bones, ulcers, diabetes
and so on. Be sure you get medical treatment when problems
arise, rather than blaming every symptom on MS.

The symptoms of MS are at least partially, temporarily manageable. The patterns of symptoms can be divided into flare-
ups, or major short-term attacks of worsening, and more
long-lasting problems that fluctuate slightly from day to day.

Flare-ups or attacks (relapses) occur frequently in MS. A
relapse is the appearance of a new neurological symptom, or
the significant worsening of old neurological symptoms, lasting
more than 24 hours and occurring without fever or acute
illness. This qualification is important, because a fever or illness
can cause latent (hidden) MS symptoms to emerge suddenly.
(Once the fever goes away, so do the symptoms.)

It was once thought that each relapse indicated the development of a new plaque of demyelination in the brain. We now

Viral infections

Among the few factors that increase the risk of a relapse are viral infections. In fact, a viral infection precedes one-quarter to one-half of all relapses. It appears that the virus triggers the relapse by provoking further action from the immune system. For this reason, if you have MS, try to avoid close contact with people who have such infections. (Typical viral infections include colds, flus and diarrheal infections such as gastroenteritis.) Also, be sure to get lots of sleep to avoid becoming run-down. When you're run-down, you're at greater risk of catching a viral infection and increasing your chance of a relapse.

Getting vaccinated against flu seems to have no effect one way or the other on your chances of having a relapse. As there are no specific antiviral treatments, the best therapy is to avoid getting viral infections in the first place.

know that only one plaque in ten produces symptoms; that is, there are ten times more plaques than there are attacks of MS. Moreover, an attack can occur because of the creation of a new plaque or the enlargement of an old plaque. Whether or not a plaque produces symptoms probably depends on where it is located in the nervous system. Plaques in the cerebral hemispheres of the brain are less likely to produce symptoms than are those in the brainstem or spinal cord. During a relapse, people with MS will develop a brand-new symptom about 20 percent of the time, and a worsening of a preexisting symptom about 80 percent of the time.

Don't confuse a relapse with a *fluctuation*, or slight change, in symptoms. A fluctuation occurs because of some factor such as stress, fatigue or emotional upset, and its severity varies directly according to how intense that factor is. When you eliminate the factor, the symptom reverts to its usual level. Fluctuations happen hour by hour, whereas flare-ups last a day or more. Fluctuations do not require treatment with steroids, nor are they evidence that your MS is "getting out of control." You manage them by dealing with whatever caused them—the stress, fatigue or emotional upset. Admittedly, it can be difficult to distinguish between a fluctuation and a relapse, but experience will usually help you tell the difference.

Relapses

Physicians classify relapses as mild, moderate and severe. These commonsense categories reflect how disabling the symptoms are. For example, new weakness in the right hand would be considered a mild relapse; new weakness in the right arm and the right leg, a moderate relapse; new weakness in the right arm and leg and great difficulty coordinating the limbs or gait, a severe relapse.

Obviously, it's best to avoid a relapse if you can. Three things will help: moderating stress, staying away from situations that worsen the MS and keeping clear of viral infections. When a relapse does occur, the first thing to do is rest more. Usually, you should stay home from work during the relapse, for at least a week to ten days. "Working through" a relapse is generally not a good idea and may indeed slow down your recovery. A relapse is not the time to get involved in strenuous physical activities. It's a time to relax and recharge your batteries.

If you are having a mild relapse, you may not need any drug therapy; it depends on how much the symptoms bother you. Over time—days, weeks, even months—the relapse usually improves. About 60 percent of people who have relapses are well on their way to recovery within eight weeks. Frequently, though, the new symptom does not disappear completely. The longer you have had MS, the less likely you are to regain your original condition after an attack. Moderate and severe relapses generally require steroid therapy, but if you wish to "ride out" the relapse, that is usually fine too.

Treating Relapses with Corticosteroids

The steroids used to treat MS relapses are potent medications with many side effects, but they have nothing to do with the anabolic steroids some athletes abuse. Steroids used in MS are *corticosteroids*, similar to the hormone *cortisol*, which the adrenal glands, situated just above the kidneys, produce. Among other things, cortisol manages the body's reaction to stresses.

Steroids are taken orally (cortisone, prednisone, decadron) or are injected intravenously (hydrocortisone, methylprednisolone). Adrenocorticotropic hormone (ACTH), which stimulates the release of cortisol, is an older medication and is not used much now.

Exactly how should steroids be administered in MS relapses? There's no simple answer. In the 1960s and early 1970s ACTH was usually injected into the muscle twice a day for about a

---

Possible side effects of steroids

Short-term use	Long-term use
• allergic reaction	• weight gain
• insomnia	• high blood pressure
• psychiatric disturbance	• cataracts
• stomach upset	• hardening of the arteries
• fluid retention	• diabetes
• increased appetite	• life-threatening infections
• acne	• osteoporosis (loss of bone mass) or other bone damage
• bone damage (rare)	• if used during pregnancy, heart defects or a cleft palate in the fetus

week. From the mid-1970s to the early 1990s, physicians usually used prednisone pills, starting at a high dose, then tapering it off over two to six weeks. During the 1980s, brief high-dose courses of steroids injected intravenously replaced the prednisone pills. In especially severe relapses, physicians may give steroids first intravenously, then orally. It's still not clear which is the best way to give steroids for relapses, or what the best dose is.

It's important to remember that although steroids *hasten* recovery from an attack of neurological symptoms in MS, they don't improve the degree of the recovery, nor do they prevent the next attack. Even if steroids are not taken, the attack will usually diminish.

Immediate possible side effects include an allergic reaction to the medication or the chemicals in which the steroid is prepared; insomnia; psychiatric disturbance; stomach upset; fluid retention; increased appetite; worsening of acne. Very rarely, bone damage termed *avascular necrosis* occurs, after even a single course of steroids.

Despite these potential problems, people usually tolerate steroids well when they are used in short courses lasting a few days or weeks. Some people even feel exuberant when on them.

Most of the side effects are manageable. A tranquilizer (sleeping pill) easily relieves insomnia. Stomach upset usually responds well to antiulcer medications such as ranitidine, taken twice a day. Except for the avascular necrosis, which damages bones permanently, the side effects can be dealt with, if necessary, by stopping the drug.

Long-term steroid use is not recommended in MS because the drugs lose their effectiveness. More important, long-term use almost always has major side effects. You gain weight,

What about relapses and...

• *immunization?*
In the past, people with MS were told that immunizations might provoke relapses. Researchers in the U.S. recently found that flu immunizations are not statistically associated with an increase or decrease in relapses; they seem to make no difference one way or the other. Every neurologist dealing with MS has his or her own opinion on this matter. Discuss it with your physician.

• *surgery?*
Most of the time, people with MS have surgery without incident, though sometimes they do have a relapse. If surgery is required, go ahead and have it without concern. There is no firm proof that surgery triggers relapses, so MS should not stop you, if the surgery is what you truly need.

• *epidural anesthesia?*
Doctors use epidurals—in which anesthetic is injected over the outer membrane of the spinal cord, called the dura—mainly during childbirth. There is no definitive evidence that epidural anesthesia worsens MS, despite long-standing concerns that it aggravates the condition. If you need an epidural, have it. If it's not necessary, don't.

particularly in the face and trunk, and look bloated. High blood pressure, cataracts, hardening of the arteries, diabetes, life-threatening infections, and osteoporosis—perhaps resulting in broken bones—may also occur. Steroid use during pregnancy may cause heart defects or a cleft palate in the fetus, but this is unusual.

People often ask physicians to prescribe long-term steroids because they "feel better" on the medication. Unfortunately, the effect is only temporary. In more advanced cases, people often notice a distinct worsening in their condition as their dose of steroids gets low or the drug is discontinued. However, once they learn the potential dangers of long-term steroid use, they are usually more comfortable staying on the drugs for no more than a few weeks at a time.

Steroids can be used more than once a year to treat relapses. Generally, the more often they are used, the less effective they become. Nonetheless, they are the cornerstone of drug treatment in MS relapses. Although researchers are exploring new drug therapies, nothing better is available yet and steroids will likely remain the mainstay of relapse treatment for some years to come. They greatly reduce the duration of suffering, and they even save lives on those rare occasions when an attack is life-threatening.

Fatigue

There are two main ways to handle the fatigue of MS: optimize your energy use, and take antifatigue medications.

The Four Ps

Energy is a precious resource that should be conserved as much as possible. Optimization of energy use involves the four Ps:

1. *Prioritization:* Do the most important activities first.
2. *Planning:* Perform necessary activities efficiently, without wasting time and/or energy.
3. *Pacing:* Work for short periods of time and then rest. How long an activity lasts should depend on your overall level of fatigue. People with MS tend to perform best after prolonged rest, so the best time of the day for them is the morning. By the end of the afternoon or the evening many are exhausted, and their performance will be much worse than first thing in the morning.
4. *Patience:* Be patient with yourself, and encourage others to be patient with you as well. Recognize that you will need more time to perform most activities, particularly those requiring sustained mental or physical exertion.

During rest times, do absolutely nothing. Making a daily or weekly schedule of activities and spreading heavy and light tasks throughout the day helps. Resting five to ten minutes every hour, for example, will allow you to function throughout the day. Every person has to determine his or her fatigue level and how best to manage it. Naturally, getting lots of sleep at night is beneficial.

Occupational therapists can help by providing advice on how to plan, how to simplify work and how to perform activities without wasting time and energy

Making Your Home Easier to Use
If you can, adapt your home to save as much of your energy as possible. The following suggestions may or may not be useful in your particular situation. They are arranged from easiest and/or least expensive to hardest and/or most expensive. Remember that your needs may fluctuate over time; these are just practical tips to help you simplify your life at home. The main thing to keep in mind is that the places where you work and relax should be as safe and comfortable as possible, and convenient enough that you do a minimum of lifting, stretching and bending.

- Access to a telephone is essential for safety and social reasons. A cordless or cellular phone carried with you eliminates the need to rush when the phone rings. Important numbers can usually be preprogrammed into the phone.
- Avoid too much clutter and crowding of furniture, so that getting around the house is easier. Floors that are smooth rather than carpeted are easier to walk on. Beware of carpet edges or high doorsills that could trip you. If you use a wheelchair or scooter much of the time, your furniture should be at a comfortable height.

- If you spend a lot of time in one room, put a small fridge or microwave oven in that room.
- If necessary, portable transfer lifts (wheeled devices that help lift you) can pick you up and put you down almost anywhere. An adjustable hospital bed is expensive but may also be useful; it makes getting in and out of bed much easier.
- Consider a ramp rather than stairs into the house. You may also want to widen doorways to accommodate a walker or wheelchair.

In the Bathroom

- Grab bars are especially useful for getting off the toilet or out of the bath. It's also easier to get off a toilet that is high— for example, one that has a commode seat placed over it.
- Showers (with curtains rather than sliding doors) are easier to get into than baths. If you do use a tub, it's useful to have a tile-covered seat at one or both ends, to help you get in or out, or for easy-to-reach storage of bath items.

In the Kitchen

- Keep the items you use most within easy reach. Peg boards provide handy storage.
- Make meals as simple and fuss-free as possible. Better yet, have someone else do the cooking.
- Make sure the level you work at is comfortable. Whenever possible, sit while you prepare meals or do the dishes.
- Sliding drawers and Lazy Susans are easier to use than deep storage bins.
- Stove controls are more easily and safely reached if they are on the front, rather than behind the cooktop. Smooth cooktops are easier to clean.

- Use a stable trolley to move sets of items such as meal settings.
- If you're using a scooter, you may find it necessary to remove the cabinet doors under the kitchen sink, and put in some sort of footrest. Even better (but more expensive), install an easy-to-get-at wall-mounted sink.

Infant and Child Care

- Don't strain your back muscles when lifting an infant or child. Hold the child close to your body. Use one arm for support if necessary. Never lift a child if you are unsteady. Be especially careful on stairs or wet floors.
- Whenever possible, care for an infant at counter height; avoid bending over or reaching.
- Use disposable diapers, as these are more convenient than reusable diapers.
- Buy clothes and shoes with Velcro fasteners; they are easier to manage than buttons or laces.
- Have an older child stand on a footstool so you can more easily help the child dress or wash.

Safety

Safety is usually a matter of common sense. Safety planning is especially important if you have problems with vision, mobility or memory.

Prevention of crime, fire and accidents should be a first goal. Under the stress of a fire or other crisis, it may be much more difficult for you to function. Ensure that you can get to and operate the phone, as well as essential doors and locks, even when you're at your worst. Ask your police and fire departments if they will do a safety inspection.

In an office

The rules for expending energy efficiently apply equally at the office. Pace yourself, taking frequent breaks as necessary. If possible, discuss the illness and its effects with your employer, and provide him or her with information on MS.

Adjust your desk and chair height to maintain proper posture and reduce slumping shoulders and neck strain. A chair with good back support is important.

Arrange the office so that file cabinets, computer terminals and so on are easily accessible. A phone device that allows the receiver to rest on your shoulder, to free your hands during extended conversations, is desirable.

A practical, well-planned and well-practiced emergency escape route is perhaps most important. It's a very good idea not to smoke at home, and to stay mindful as to whether the stove is turned off, the doors are locked and so on.

Peepholes are relatively inexpensive, and let you see who is at the door before you decide whether to open it. An intercom system at the door is another solution. It's wise not to open the door to strangers, especially if you are alone.

Every home needs smoke detectors; check the system weekly and change the batteries regularly (see the manufacturer's instructions). You should also have a carbon monoxide detector.

If you have a lot of trouble with dizziness or with getting around, you may want to wear a personal alarm around your neck, to alert family or a monitoring company that you need help. You might consider getting a trained service dog to assist in opening doors, fetching items and giving physical and emotional support.

Medications to Manage Fatigue

A number of medications help to relieve the symptoms of fatigue in MS. Only about half the people taking these drugs gain enough relief to justify using them on a long-term basis. The medications work best to treat the overwhelming fatigue and lassitude of MS. They do not eliminate normal feelings of tiredness. It's always best to try to sort out the cause of your exhaustion—true MS-related fatigue, reduced endurance, masked depression or simply the normal weariness everyone experiences at the end of a hard day—before taking any drugs.

Modafinil, originally developed to treat the sleeping disorder of narcolepsy, has recently been found effective against MS-related fatigue. Although it does not help everyone, it does help many people, and it is my first choice for this purpose. Side effects are mild but may include feeling "jittery."

Amantadine increases dopamine levels in the brain. Dopamine is a chemical that facilitates communication between nerve cells. Precisely why it works in MS is unknown, but it appears to be a mild general stimulant. Some people complain of difficulty sleeping when using the medication. It has other potential side effects, although these are relatively uncommon and generally do not cause significant difficulty.

Methylphenidate is another amphetamine. Physicians use it to treat attention deficit disorder or obesity. It is potentially addictive and, because it is a powerful stimulant, it may have undesirable effects on blood pressure and heart function, although the vast majority of people who take it report no significant side effects. Modafinil and methylphenidate may cause insomnia—their most common side effect.

More recently, physicians have used antidepressant medications such as *fluoxetine* to treat the fatigue of some MS sufferers. This again raises the question of whether at least some of what people call fatigue is actually depression.

Pain

Many people believe that MS is a painless disease. In fact, at least 20 to 50 percent of those with MS report significant pain. They get all the pains that other folks get, of course, but they also get pains that specifically indicate a neurological problem. These pains result from short circuits in the neuron pathways that carry electrical impulses in the brain and spinal cord.

Trigeminal neuralgia, also known as *tic douloureux*, is a stabbing facial pain. It is excruciating, although it lasts for only seconds to minutes. In MS, it often goes away on its own after a few months. Medications to dull the pain include *gabapentin, carbamazepine, phenytoin* and *baclofen* (although baclofen is used more commonly for limb stiffness). These medications calm the short circuits causing the pain. All four have a sedative effect, so each must be started at a low dose and slowly increased to a dose that adequately controls the pain. If they don't work, a surgical procedure called a *percutaneous rhizotomy* is done under local anesthesia, in which the surgeon cuts the nerve causing the pain. It helps most people, but it produces numbness in the face, so physicians use it only as a last resort.

Another pain seen in MS is Lhermitte's sign. Here, pain shoots down the spine into the arms or legs when the person flexes his or her neck. The brief sensation is more disturbing than discomforting. It indicates a problem in the neck area of the spine. Although it can appear at any time in MS, it frequently occurs early in the illness.

Dysesthesia is a burning, aching, tingling discomfort that occurs most commonly in the limbs. It is treated with gabapentin, carbamazepine and phenytoin. Alternatively, a low dose of the antidepressant *amitriptyline* often helps. Creams containing irritants such as capsaicin, which you rub into the skin, are somewhat useful, although they substitute one burning sensation for another. Transcutaneous electrical nerve stimulation (TENS), which involves mild electrical stimulation of the painful area, can be tried. The machine that delivers the stimulus is small, portable and relatively inexpensive. Other pain management techniques include biofeedback, meditation and acupuncture (see later in this chapter). They are highly variable in their effectiveness, and predicting who will and will not respond is difficult.

Standard painkillers such as acetylsalicylic acid or ASA (called aspirin in the U.S.), codeine, acetaminophen, anti-inflammatory drugs and narcotics are also highly variable in their effectiveness, although they do afford some relief. Narcotics must always be used carefully because they are addictive but they are sometimes necessary when all else fails.

Low back pain is common in people with MS, but MS itself does not cause low back pain. It also does not cause pain or swelling in the joints. Pain in the back or joints sometimes occurs because of an altered way of walking or standing that puts extra stress on these areas. Heavy lifting and inappropriate turning and bending in people who are already weak may also be factors. These movements may irritate the spinal nerves or even cause a disc to slip. Heat massage and ultrasound frequently help this kind of pain, as well as exercises designed to relieve spasms of the back muscle. Drugs, including *cyclobenzaprine* and *methocarbamol*, may also be used.

Naturally, proper treatment of any type of pain depends on correct diagnosis of its cause. Having pain in MS does not, in itself, indicate that the disease is getting worse.

The marijuana debate

What about using marijuana to treat MS symptoms such as pain, spasticity or tremor? Although not enough research has been done in this area, it appears to me that some patients do obtain relief from these symptoms by smoking marijuana. However, they may also become intoxicated ("high"), and the long-term safety of the drug is unclear. If marijuana is used it should be as a last resort, under close medical supervision, and in accordance with local laws.

Bladder Problems

Normal voiding (emptying) of the bladder depends on proper functioning of the pathways between the brain and the voiding reflex center (VRC), which is located at the base of the spinal cord. When the bladder is full, it is sufficiently stretched to stimulate nerves in the bladder wall. These nerves signal the VRC, which in turn signals the brain, and you become aware of the need to urinate. The brain either signals the VRC and, in turn, the urethral sphincter (the muscle that regulates the flow of urine out of the body) that it's okay to go ahead, or tells it to contract so that you can wait. In MS these nerve pathways may be damaged. The location of the damage will determine the kind of bladder problem you have, and the kind of bladder problem you have will determine the treatment. In MS there are three kinds of bladder dysfunction.

Spastic Small Bladder

The most common problem is a spastic small bladder, sometimes called a *disinhibited* bladder. It results from demyelination of the pathways between the VRC and the brain. The question of whether or not to empty the bladder is no longer under voluntary control, and voiding (urination) becomes a reflex reaction to the "filling" signal. This type of bladder produces symptoms of urinary frequency, urgency, dribbling and/or incontinence. The bladder remains small because, as soon as it starts to fill, it empties.

Urinary system

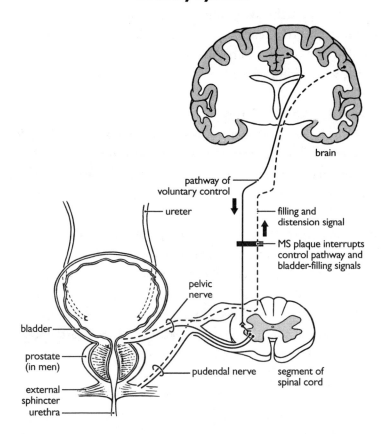

Flaccid Big Bladder

If demyelination occurs in the area of the VRC, a flaccid or *inhibited* bladder may result. The bladder fills with urine but communications to or from the VRC have been cut, so the bladder doesn't receive the command to empty. The bladder becomes overfilled and stretched. This produces symptoms of urinary frequency, urgency, dribbling, hesitancy and incontinence. Because urine stays in the bladder longer than it ought to, the bladder is prone to infection.

Notice that the symptoms of either small or big bladder dysfunction (frequency, urgency, dribbling, incontinence) are similar, so it is not possible to tell, simply on the basis of symptoms, which kind of bladder dysfunction is present.

Incoordinated Bladder
The third type of bladder problem is the incoordinated bladder (a fancier name is *detrusor sphincter dyssynergia*). Here, either the sphincter remains closed when the bladder wall contracts, creating a sense of urgency followed by hesitancy in voiding, or the bladder wall relaxes while the sphincter stays open, causing dribbling, incontinence and overfilling of the bladder. This too is due to demyelination in the region of the VRC or elsewhere, resulting in a lack of coordination between the sphincter and the bladder wall. The bladder is usually either spastic or flaccid.

Despite these bladder problems, kidney diseases are uncommon in MS. However, bladder infections, which sometimes spread to the kidneys and even the blood, occur frequently and require prompt investigation and appropriate treatment, including antibiotics. People with MS can become very ill from urine infections, which may in turn trigger relapses.

Treating Bladder Problems
The first step in managing bladder problems in MS is to determine which kind of bladder problem you have. A key way is

to find out how much urine remains in the bladder after voiding. If there is a lot (more than 150 cc), you have a flaccid big bladder; if there is less than 100 cc, you have a normal or a small spastic bladder. An incoordinated bladder may contain either more or less than 150 cc.

The spastic small bladder is best treated with medications that "slow" the bladder—that is, that decrease the transmission of impulses from the VRC that cause it to empty. These include *oxybutynin, tolterodine, propantheline, flavoxate* and *imipramine*. They lengthen the intervals between urinations and decrease the sense of urgency, giving you more time to reach the bathroom and to avoid dribbling and incontinence.

The flaccid big bladder cannot usually be treated just with medication. In mild cases, a method that helps you to empty the bladder more completely is the *Credé maneuver* of bladder massage. After you've voided as much urine as possible naturally, you apply downward pressure to the lower abdomen with both hands while bearing down. This technique can be performed only when you're sitting, which requires a change in behavior for men.

If the bladder cannot be emptied sufficiently using the Credé maneuver, intermittent self-catheterization may be necessary. A small tube (catheter) is inserted through the urethra (the canal through which urine is discharged) into the bladder to allow the urine to drain. This is much easier to do than it sounds, and it poses very little risk of damage, particularly in women, who tend to have a short urethra. There is, however, some risk of infection. It enables you to decide when to empty the bladder, and thus avoid dribbling or incontinence. How often should this be done? Timing varies from person to person, but usually it need not be done more than about every four to six hours. Medications such as oxybutynin are sometimes used with self-catheterization, to relax the bladder and allow it to fill more completely and to decrease dribbling and incontinence between catheterizations. Self-catheterization also allows a stretched bladder wall to gradually shrink back to normal size and, sometimes, function.

The problem with self-catheterization is that you have to have sufficient arm control to insert the tube into the bladder. If you don't, continuous catheterization with a Foley catheter may be necessary. It is inserted into the bladder and connected to a collecting bag. As urine goes into the bladder, it drains out the catheter into the bag. Chronic use of a Foley catheter carries a significant risk of urinary tract infections, so physicians insert it only when absolutely necessary. A permanent in-dwelling catheter has to be changed about once every month by a nurse. A condom catheter—which fits over the penis, like a condom, and is connected by a tube to a collecting bag—may be useful for men, but it will help only if the bladder empties itself automatically. The penis must be big enough for the condom to stick to the shaft. Because of dampness and friction, care must be taken not to ulcerate the penis. Unfortunately, female condom catheters tend to fall off, and to date are not reliable enough for use.

An uncoordinated bladder may result in either too little or too much urine left in the bladder after urination. If too much urine remains (residual urine), catheterization will be necessary. If there is too little urine, bladder-inhibiting medication such as oxybutynin, propantheline, flavoxate or imipramine will be necessary.

Significant bladder symptoms require a urological assessment. This is known as "urodynamic testing." It is simple to perform and is relatively safe. The examination may be combined with a cystoscopy, in which the urologist inserts a small telescope into the bladder to look at the walls. This can show whether the bladder is too small or too big.

Occasionally, medications called *alpha blockers* help an incoordinated bladder. Alpha blockers were originally developed to treat high blood pressure, but they can also help the bladder work in a slightly more coordinated fashion. *Clonidine* and *terazosin* are alpha blockers that are sometimes used to try to improve coordination and increase bladder control.

Some people lose urine mainly at night, while sleeping. A new hormone medication called *desmopressin* mimics a brain hormone that decreases urine formation in the kidneys and

Tips for preventing bladder infections

- Empty the bladder completely, using self-catheterization techniques if necessary. Make the urine more acidic by drinking cranberry juice or taking high doses of vitamin C (1,000 to 4,000 mg a day), to retard bacterial growth. If you have a history of urinary tract infections, ask your physician about low-dose antibiotics.

- Avoid holding urine in the bladder for long periods.

- If you're a woman, be careful to wipe from front to back, especially after a bowel movement, and avoid undergarments made of synthetic materials—they tend to trap moisture, which encourages the growth of bacteria.

- If you're a woman and have recurrent bladder infections, empty the bladder both before and after intercourse to flush away any bacteria.

- Drink adequate amounts of fluid to keep the bladder flushed, generally eight to twelve glasses a day.

- If you have an in-dwelling Foley catheter, keep the tubing and drainage bag as clean as possible. Change the catheter at least once a month, using proper sterile techniques.

- If you have urinary symptoms, seek medical attention. Urinary tract infections can pose a serious threat to health if left untreated. Many relapses of MS occur during or after urinary infections.

- When you have a urinary tract infection and your physician prescribes antibiotics, take them as directed, for the full time indicated, to ensure that all invading bacteria are destroyed. If you stop early because you're feeling better, any remaining bacteria will re-invade and cause problems again.

therefore lowers the probability of waking up in a wet bed. It is most convenient as a nasal spray. Other people benefit from imipramine or oxybutynin taken just before bed, to let the bladder fill up more at night.

Urinary Tract (Bladder) Infections

Urinary tract infections are common in MS for a variety of reasons. The flaccid bladder fails to empty completely and bacteria grow in the remaining urine. Intermittent self-catheterization may introduce bacteria into the bladder, producing infection. An in-dwelling Foley catheter provides bacteria with a route to the bladder. Women have a shorter urethra than men and are more prone to develop bladder infection because bacteria can reach the bladder more easily.

A urine culture confirms the diagnosis of urinary tract infection. You collect some urine in a sterile bottle and the lab then tests for bacteria. The presence of bacteria does not mean that the infection requires treatment—anyone with an in-dwelling Foley catheter will test positive for bacteria. But antibiotic treatment is called for when there is urinary frequency or urgency, burning or discomfort when urinating, fever or foul-smelling urine. Blood or mucus in the urine also suggests the need for treatment. Physicians usually prescribe an oral antibiotic which you take for seven to ten days. Intravenous antibiotics are necessary only for severe infections accompanied by fever and malaise.

Bowel Problems

Many people with MS have bowel difficulties, although they are usually less worrisome than bladder problems. The main symptoms are constipation and diarrhea.

Constipation

Constipation is the infrequent or difficult elimination of stool. It is the most common bowel problem in MS. Eliminating stools is analogous to urinary voiding. When the rectum, which constitutes the last five or six inches (12 to 15 cm) of gastrointestinal tract, fills with stool, a "filled" signal is sent to the brain. If the time is appropriate, the external sphincter of the anus relaxes so a bowel movement can occur. If the time is not appropriate, the external sphincter constricts to delay the bowel movement. As in urination, relaxation of the external sphincter is what sets the process in motion.

Constipation occurs in MS because demyelination in the brain or spinal cord interferes with nerve messages to the bowel. In addition, someone with MS may limit his or her fluid intake because of bladder difficulties; because the body requires water, it will then be absorbed from the stool as the stool passes through the colon. This loss of water results in hard, compact stool. As well, weakness, spasticity or fatigue may significantly limit physical activity, which in turn slows bowel activity and causes constipation. Some medicines taken for other problems such as bladder frequency or depression may also slow the bowel.

How to Manage Constipation

- Drink adequate amounts of liquid (8 to 12 glasses daily).
- Add fiber to your diet. It softens the stool and decreases the amount of time required for the stool to pass through the intestinal tract. Sources include whole-grain breads and cereals, fruits and vegetables, nuts, seeds and beans. But don't incorporate high-fiber foods too quickly or they may produce gas and, occasionally, diarrhea. Start them in small amounts and increase your intake over time.

High-fiber foods help constipation
For a healthy bowel, include in your daily diet:
- one serving of fruit (with the skin left on) or vegetable, cooked, raw or dried
- one-half to one serving of whole wheat or rye bread or fruit juice
- one serving (1 tablespoon/15 mL) of bran, nuts or seeds. Eat raw bran plain, or mixed with cereal, applesauce, soups, yogurt or casseroles; or add it to flour in cooking or baking.

- Train your bowels. Select the time that is most convenient for having a bowel movement—usually shortly after a meal, since the bowel is normally more active then. Drink a cup of hot or lukewarm coffee, tea or water; it frequently encourages a bowel movement. Schedule fifteen to twenty minutes of uninterrupted time daily for this activity, and stick to the routine, even if it proves difficult initially.
- Ask your doctor about medications for constipation. There is a long list, ranging from mild bulk-forming agents based on fiber, through stronger oral stimulants like milk of magnesia, to suppositories and rectal stimulants (enemas).

Diarrhea and Incontinence
Occasionally, diarrhea (loose, frequent bowel movements) is a problem. A bulk-forming agent may help firm up the stool. Drink fluids as necessary. If the problem persists, treatment with *loperamide* may help. Otherwise, see your doctor.

From time to time you may have trouble with bowel urgency and even incontinence—that is, not being able to reach a toilet in time. Obviously this can be extremely distressing. It tends to happen infrequently, however, and is managed by developing a bowel routine (a regular "time to go"). If this isn't enough, an agent such as oxybutynin may be used, to decrease the bowel spasms that are causing the problem.

Depression, Anxiety and Stress

Depression

If you have MS, you have many good reasons to feel depressed: MS does not end your life, but the resulting uncertainty about your future can make life hard to enjoy. You may experience a loss in self-esteem, and changes in self-image, life plans, goals and values; you may fear rejection by family and friends. Financial implications can also be very negative.

Depression in MS arises as a reaction to negative circumstances and experiences associated with the disease (*reactive depression*), or as the result of changes in the frontal and temporal lobes of the brain, as well as the emotional part of the brain, called the limbic system (*endogenous depression*). In real life, though, it is rarely clear how much of the depression is from direct physical causes, and how much is emotional in origin. Treatment is the same in either case.

The good news about depression is that it is highly treatable. First, you need a counselor—usually a family physician,

Grieving

When you find out you have MS, you may go through a grieving process similar to what you would experience with any major loss. In writing about bereavement, Elisabeth Kübler-Ross described five stages of grieving: denial, anger, bargaining, depression and acceptance.

However, not every person begins at denial and proceeds step by step to acceptance. The order of the stages may vary from person to person, and you may jump from one stage to another and back. Perhaps it's more accurate to consider denial, anger, bargaining, depression and acceptance as five different ways of coping with a major loss. On some days you use denial; on others, anger; on yet others, bargaining. None is necessarily "better." It all depends on the circumstances. In any case, such feelings are part of a normal, healthy adjustment to your new situation. Don't feel guilty if you find yourself cycling back and forth through these various moods.

psychiatrist, psychologist or social worker in whom you have confidence. This counselor must be willing to let you express your emotions, fully and openly, over time. "Talk therapy" is an important part of dealing with depression.

Medications also play a significant role. In the past, depression was treated with tricyclic antidepressants such as amitriptyline, nortriptyline or imipramine. Nowadays physicians generally prescribe the newer class of antidepressants known as SSRIs (selective serotonin re-uptake inhibitors). They are easier to use than tricyclic antidepressants, because they have fewer, milder side effects, and they are very effective, and safer to use. Even newer classes of antidepressants will be available soon.

Although all antidepressants have slightly different side effects, in general the tricyclics cause drowsiness and dry mouth. The newer SSRI antidepressants usually cause temporary drowsiness and decreased sex drive. Weight gain can occur with either tricyclic antidepressants or SSRIs, although it's more common with tricyclics. Dosage with either type of drug usually "begins low and goes slow"; the amount taken is gradually increased over weeks to months as necessary. In most cases, it takes at least a month before you see results from antidepressant treatment. And if you don't respond to one antidepressant, you may well respond to another in the same class. There are many different antidepressants, and new classes are constantly being developed, with fewer side effects such as sedation and decreased libido. Chances are excellent that one or more will work for you. But predicting who will respond to which medication is impossible and, as with most medications, treatment is essentially trial and error.

Anxiety

Depression in MS is often mixed with increased feelings of anxiety, especially soon after the diagnosis. It too may be reactive (an emotional response to all the other problems) or endogenous (a result of physical changes in the brain). Anxiety can be treated with tranquilizers and sometimes with antidepressants, together with supportive counseling. Drugs used to treat anxiety include *lorazepam* and *buspirone*, as well as some of the antidepressants.

Occasionally, MS causes emotional instability. Episodes of crying and laughing often follow each other from minute to minute. People lose control emotionally, and often find it embarrassing. This is called "pathological laughter and crying." It results from demyelination or "short-circuiting" in the frontal lobe of the brain. Antidepressants such as amitriptyline help to restore the ability to maintain emotional equilibrium.

Stress

By "stress" we usually mean emotional tension that shows up as anxiety, poor concentration and poor problem solving, although stress can also manifest itself physically, in abdominal cramps, diarrhea, headaches, muscle spasms, neck pain, increased blood pressure and pulse rate, fatigue and insomnia. Can stress be bad for you if you have MS? Does it trigger relapses or worsen your prognosis? Studies looking at this important question have had contradictory results. Though we do know that stress does not *cause* MS, it's wise to avoid extreme stress with this condition. People with MS often have relapses after major emotional traumas such as a marital breakup, the loss of a loved one or a major illness in a child.

Workplace stress, too, appears to contribute to an increase in relapses, particularly where the stress is extreme and persistent. Stress certainly makes the symptoms of MS *feel* worse, and this may contribute to the perception that it causes relapses. Common sense says it's advisable to minimize emotional upheaval in your life when you have MS. Whether stress itself causes your MS to worsen is an open question.

Physical Stress

Sometimes the cause of stress is physical rather than emotional. If you find that heat worsens your symptoms (Uhthoff's phenomenon), just avoid getting overheated. However, not all people with MS have a problem with heat; many enjoy the warmth of the summer, or visits to warmer countries, without any worsening of symptoms. There is *no* proof that heat can trigger a relapse, although some neurologists believe that it can. Heat, including a fever, simply uncovers the problems that were already there; it does not create new symptoms, or cause new damage in the nervous system. In fact, some people find that cold worsens their symptoms, particularly muscle stiffness and cramping. The best course of action is to avoid any temperature stress that makes things worse.

From time to time people will say they've had a relapse after a motor vehicle accident. Perhaps because of the legal implications, scientists have probed this claim. Several studies have tried to determine whether a severe physical stress increases the risk of a relapse. The answer is probably no. Physical stress—a whiplash injury in a car accident, falling on the sidewalk and breaking a bone—neither causes MS nor increases the risk of a relapse. Again, association is not the same thing as causation. Although people sometimes have relapses after

Strategies for coping with stress

Many people with MS don't recognize the psychological component of their condition at first, and only gradually accept the fact that they may need to develop coping strategies. These include learning how to deal effectively with the new issues confronting them: stereotypes of the disabled in the community, perceived changes in masculinity or femininity, changes in relationships, changes in roles within the family, changes in employment status, increased dependence on others and changes in physical condition. Coping strategies are best developed through experience; they cannot be learned by reading a book. But here are a few strategies to get you started:

- Foster the idea of being in control. Focus on the many aspects of your life in which you do have control, such as what you do today, whom you socialize with and so on. To be happy and to cope, people must feel that they have at least some—preferably a lot of—control over their lives.
- Determine a way (small or large) to contribute to your community—something you can enjoy—and follow through with your plan. This will enhance your self-esteem and help put your problems in perspective.
- Attend appropriate counseling sessions.
- Learn to say no without feeling guilty.
- Make a list of people, places and things you like (energizers) and dislike (fatiguers). Be honest. Within the limits of your ethical responsibilities, avoid fatiguers and seek out energizers.
- Make a list of people you can rely on for support, and call on them as needed. Create support networks outside the home (where most of the support is ordinarily provided).
- Prioritize projects to avoid burnout and overload.

A spouse, close friend, religious adviser, counselor or physician who listens with empathy can help you cope better. It's difficult to deal with MS in isolation from others. Your local multiple sclerosis society can probably provide information on support resources in your area (see Further Resources, at the end of this book).

car accidents, they also have relapses after watching their favorite television show.

Some people rely on relaxation techniques to control stress; others find prayer relaxing. Some find a hot bath or music helpful; for others, it's watching TV. Whatever relaxes you is a stress-management tool. Be leery of self-help gurus who promise new and exotic relaxation techniques. (See Alternative Therapies, later in this chapter.) If you've found a way to relax, you're already there.

Stress counseling, done individually or in a group, may also help. By understanding the stress that accompanies a chronic disease, you can achieve a healthier mental state. The physical changes of MS sometimes lead to emotional challenges, but these can be dealt with through patience, perseverance and support from others.

Exercise

Of paramount interest to many people with MS is exercise—which is a very real physical stress. Research indicates that *moderate* exercise increases their feeling of well-being and self-confidence, and also improves—albeit modestly—strength and cardiovascular conditioning. In a study from Utah, 54 people with MS who exercised aerobically on a stationary bike over a 15-week period showed an increase in cardiovascular fitness and muscle strength, as well as reduced levels of depression, anger and their usual fatigue. In another study, from the University of Washington, 8 women with MS who lifted weights over 12 weeks showed improved ability to perform everyday tasks such as walking up stairs. Since both these studies followed small groups of people over a short time, the results are preliminary and must be interpreted with caution. They do suggest, though, that regular exercise has both physical and psychological benefits for people with MS.

There are different types of exercise that may help. In *range-of-motion exercises*, the arms and legs are moved through the full range of the joints' motion, to prevent muscle shortening and contractures (joint immobilization). If necessary, get someone to assist you with these stretching exercises. *Aerobic exercise*—such as walking, stationary bicycling and swimming—may also be useful. Consult your neurologist before deciding what's best for you.

Try to avoid getting overheated during exercise; a cool bath before and after helps, or swimming in a cool pool rather than a warm one. You can buy special cooling vests, but they are rather costly (U.S. $300 to $1000, depending on the options you want).

A physiotherapist can advise you on your exercise program, both before you start and as you progress, and the feedback you get may help you stick with the program.

How far should you go? To the point of fatigue but not exhaustion. If you are more than usually tired the day after exercise, you've gone too far. The more advanced your MS, the more moderate the exercise should be.

Of course, there is great psychological benefit in feeling that, by exercising, you are taking charge of your health and doing something good for yourself. On the other hand, overestimating the benefits of exercise may lead to disappointment and a feeling of failure. Moderate exercise is a good thing but it will not determine whether you have "good, medium or bad" MS. Keep moving, but don't overdo it.

Memory Problems

Cognitive neurorehabilitation is a fancy term for strategies that help you improve your memory or use it better. Before starting, remember that memory is complex. Not only does the disease process itself worsen memory, but so do stress, anxiety, fatigue and depression, because they impair your ability to concentrate. If you can't concentrate, you won't be able to remember, whether you have MS or not.

Here are some strategies that can help with memory problems.

- Make lists! They are the best memory enhancers for anyone.
- Jot down appointments and special days on a calendar.
- Log daily events, reminders, messages from family and friends in a notebook of "things to remember."
- Use a tape recorder to help remember information.
- Write down *immediately* the things you need to remember.
- Keep home and work organized and put things back where they're supposed to go. That way, you'll know where to look for them.

Some people report improved cognition with the use of pemoline or methylphenidate. But these drugs treat the fatigue rather than any cognitive difficulties. Most of the time they are not helpful when the main problem is memory itself, rather than fatigue. For this reason, they are not usually recommended.

Preliminary evidence suggests that treatment over time with interferon beta (see Chapter Six) may slow cognitive deterioration in MS. However, this finding requires further confirmation. It would be nice if a "smart pill" existed. We'd all want to use it!

Spasticity (Muscle Stiffness)

Muscles work in groups; with most movements, two groups of muscles act simultaneously on a joint. Normally, when muscles in one group contract, the opposing muscle group relaxes. This allows smooth, coordinated movement. In MS, this delicate balance is disrupted. Opposing groups of muscles contract simultaneously. The result is constant stiffness, called "spasticity." Spasms—painful cramplike muscle contractions—are often associated with spasticity, but spasms and spasticity are *not* the same thing.

Spasticity usually occurs in the antigravity, or postural, muscles—the larger, stronger muscles responsible for maintaining our upright posture and/or moving against gravity. These include the gastrocnemius muscles of the calf, the quadriceps at the front of the thigh, and the adductor in the groin, as well as the biceps in the upper arm and the pronator in the forearm, among others.

Increased stiffness means that performing everyday activities requires a great deal of work. Reducing spasticity means greater freedom of movement and, frequently, less fatigue. Often, the limbs are both weak and spastic. However, the one good thing about spasticity is that this stiffening of a limb can help compensate for weakness. For example, it's easier to stand on a weak leg if the muscles are stiff. Reducing or eliminating spasticity through drugs or other treatments can unmask weakness, causing more trouble than benefit and interfering with the person's already limited ability to get around.

There are a variety of ways to treat spasticity.

Stretching
One simple way is to stretch the muscles that are spastic. Hold the stretch for about a minute, then ease off. Contact your local multiple sclerosis society for resources on this subject. Or consult a physiotherapist; he or she will tailor an exercise program to meet your needs.

Exercising in a pool may be extremely beneficial because the buoyancy of the water allows you to move spastic limbs more freely. The coolness of the water also helps many people with MS find partial relief of their symptoms. Use the pool to do both stretching and the easy, slow, rhythmic calisthenics of range-of-motion exercises. Avoid an excessively warm pool; it may produce fatigue. How warm is too warm? Probably anything over 80 degrees Fahrenheit (26 degrees Celsius).

No scientific study has ever shown that stretching produces a pronounced or long-lasting effect. But most physiotherapists and neurologists believe that it relieves spasticity at least temporarily. Progressively relaxing a muscle as you breathe deeply and visualize the muscle may also help, particularly in milder cases of spasticity.

Relaxation
Stress exacerbates spasticity. Relaxation helps you control spasticity better by putting you more in control of your well-being. To be successful at it, you must learn to let go of thoughts that drift in and out of your mind. Practice the following steps until they become second nature.

1. Find a quiet place where you can be on your own for 20 or 30 minutes.
2. Sit with your arms, head and feet supported, or lie down.
3. Close your eyes. Focus on your breathing. The goal is to breathe deeply, slowly and evenly. Music may help.
4. Systematically relax your muscles, working up from your feet. First tell your feet to relax, then your calves, thighs, buttocks, abdomen, chest, arms, hands, neck and head.
5. Let your body feel heavier and heavier with each breath, as though it is sinking into the floor.
6. Imagine yourself in a place you have always wanted to go to, or return to. Think of the sights, sounds and smells. Try to enjoy the place with all your senses.

7. When you are ready to leave, go with the knowledge that you can return at will. Open your eyes slowly and try to carry the feeling of relaxation back into your normal world.

This relaxation technique may help you deal with many other symptoms of MS as well, such as anxiety, fatigue and depression.

Medications

Baclofen is the cornerstone of antispasticity drug therapy in MS, and most people respond well to it. Baclofen calms nerves in the spinal cord. However, the dose must be carefully determined. Usually, physicians arrive at the correct dosage by starting off at a low dose and slowly increasing it until they obtain the maximum beneficial effect. Taking too much initially produces weakness and fatigue. The person then abandons the drug because of its side effects, never having taken it long enough to enjoy the relief it can provide. The correct dose is highly variable, ranging from 5 mg to 80 mg a day. Most people take baclofen in pill form. Other than weakness or fatigue, serious side effects are uncommon with the pill.

There are also experimental ways of providing this medication, such as through a pump implanted under the skin of the abdomen and connected directly to the lower half of the spinal-cord area. This is technically difficult, and necessary only in the most severe cases of spasticity. As with any invasive procedure, the risks are greater, as are the costs. Nonetheless, administering baclofen this way produces dramatic effects in some cases where spasticity pills have not worked.

Medications for spasticity are particularly useful when people already use a wheelchair most of the time, and are having difficulty with arm stiffness or leg spasms. These leg spasms can be quite painful, and because they often occur at night, they interfere with sleep.

Tizanidine is a fairly new drug for the treatment of spasticity. It is quite effective, less sedating than baclofen and the benzodiazepines, and may cause slightly less weakness than other medications, although this remains to be firmly established. Baclofen and tizanidine are the two most useful drugs for MS-related spasticity.

Although best known as tranquilizers, members of the benzodiazepine family (such as diazepam and lorazepam) also relieve spasticity and spasms. However, they cause drowsiness and weakness and are generally not that useful on a day-to-day basis. They are potentially addictive, as well.

Physicians sometimes prescribe *dantrolene* for spasticity. It acts directly on muscle cells and can be helpful, but it frequently produces a feeling of increased weakness. It may damage the liver, so it isn't a first-choice treatment.

The prescribing physician should closely monitor the use of any of these drugs. If you decide to go off any of them, taper off over a week or two or longer, rather than stopping abruptly. Withdrawing suddenly, particularly if you have used these drugs for a long time (weeks to months), may cause seizures. Discuss how to stop these medications with your physician.

Some people with MS develop sudden cramps called *tonic spasms*. Here, an entire arm or leg draws itself into a stiff, flexed or extended position. Most people who suffer from these spasms also have underlying spasticity. In some instances, tonic spasms are strong, worrying and painful. They respond well to low doses of gabapentin, carbamazepine or phenytoin. Untreated, they can last for a few minutes at a time.

Mechanical Aids

Devices can be made up to counteract spasticity and prevent *contracture*, in which a joint loses its range of movement or becomes "locked." For example, splints spread the fingers or toes and aid in mobility or limb function. Braces can keep a wrist, foot or hand in a neutral position and prevent deformity or help in movement. These devices are known as *orthoses* or *orthotics*.

Injection Therapy

Occasionally, stretching, relaxation, medications and mechanical aids all fail to relieve spasticity. At this point it is time to consider injection therapy. There are two options.

A new injection treatment uses *botulin*, a toxin produced by the bacteria that causes botulism, an often fatal food poisoning. When small amounts of botulin are injected into a muscle where the nerves join it, temporary paralysis results. This relieves the spasticity. Physicians use botulin mostly for spasms in the thigh, but it can also be used for spasms in the eye or face, or to reduce wrinkles. The effects of botulin wear off after a few months, with no irreversible damage. On the other hand, you will need repeated injections, and these may become costly for either you or your insurance company. Where feasible, botulin injections are preferable to the other option, *phenol* injection.

Phenol is injected into the nerves producing the unwanted muscle activity. The chemical damages or destroys the nerves and the muscle becomes flaccid (limp). The procedure is not without risks. The precise risks depend on the location of the injection. If phenol is injected into nerves for the leg muscles, there may be temporary loss of bowel and bladder control. Make sure you ask your physician about the risks before consenting to this treatment.

Surgery

Surgical procedures for spasticity involve cutting nerves or tendons so that muscles cannot contract and go into spasm. These operations are rarely required, but in some instances, particularly with leg spasticity, they provide dramatic relief.

Weakness

Weakness is one of the most disabling symptoms of MS. The first step in treating it is to sort out whether it comes from simple disuse of the muscle, fatigue or true neurological paralysis. If a muscle is weak because it has not been used, exercise will strengthen it. If it is weak due to fatigue, rest will help. However, if it is weak because of poorly transmitted electrical impulses in the brain or spinal cord, exercise will not help much. Think of a lightbulb that flickers on and off because of a loose connection. In MS the problem is a "loose connection" between the brain and spinal cord and the muscle itself. Just as turning the light on and off will not make it work better, no amount of exercise will eliminate neurological muscle weakness.

At this point, we have no medication to reverse weakness. However, a new class of drugs known as potassium channel blockers holds some promise. Early trials are somewhat encouraging, despite worrisome side effects of dizziness and occasional seizures. The hope is that subsequent testing of this type of medication will identify an agent that both safely and effectively reverses neurological weakness.

Problems in Walking

Difficulty walking is a major problem in MS. Spasticity, reduced endurance, weakness and imbalance all impair normal walking. Not being able to walk is the most visible sign of disability, and the most typical problem faced by people with long-standing or more advanced MS.

Our ability to be mobile is central to our perception of the quality of our lives. Obviously, impaired walking can make daily life more difficult, at work, at home and traveling between the two. If your walking becomes impaired, use one of the aids described below to help you stay mobile and independent, and use it without delay. Using an aid isn't the same as walking unassisted, of course, but it is surely better than the practical problems that can come with losing your mobility and independence.

Braces

If only part of your leg is weak, such as the foot or knee, specially created braces can allow for reasonably normal leg function. Naturally, wearing sensible shoes is important. They should have a nonslippery sole and be low-heeled. If you have a drop foot (caused by paralysis of the front leg muscles), use an ankle-foot orthotic, known as an AFO. It permits the foot to move more normally during walking. If the knee tends to collapse or become hyperextended during walking, use a brace over that joint.

Canes

Except for localized kinds of weakness, orthotics and braces are not that useful. Particularly when poor balance accompanies more advanced weakness, people will benefit more from assistive devices such as canes and crutches. There is absolutely nothing wrong with using them, and no one should feel weak-willed in relying on them. They are simply commonsense tools to improve mobility.

Many people with permanent unsteadiness or staggering use a cane when walking. You usually carry a cane in the hand opposite the weak leg. Walking involves "reciprocal movement"—the left hand goes forward when the right foot goes forward and vice versa. The cane precedes or accompanies the weak leg; it does not follow it. If weakness is pronounced in both legs you may need two canes, although a walker is typically used in that case. With two canes the same walking pattern applies; the left foot and the right hand go forward together, then the right foot and the left hand. Walking this way is slower, but balance and stability increase. When walking up the stairs, step up with the strong leg first. When descending, step down with the weak leg first. "Go up with the good and down with the bad," so that the strong leg does all the work of lifting and lowering you. Again, the cane should accompany or precede the weak leg. If a handrail is available, use it.

Crutches

Forearm crutches (braced against the forearms, instead of in the armpits) provide more stability than a standard cane, although they appear more cumbersome. Crutches require less strength in the arms than do canes, and are more stable. They are recommended if your balance and strength are more severely affected.

Walkers and Wheelchairs

Many walkers have brakes and carrying baskets and are quite elaborate. They are often on wheels. Use the same walking pattern as with a cane. Walk forward with the walker at arm's length ahead, putting your strong leg forward first, then your weak leg. Take normal steps. If walking is still extremely difficult or impossible, a wheelchair may be the correct choice. Don't be afraid to use one; it's just another tool to increase your mobility. Many types are available. A standard manual wheelchair may not provide you with enough independence, because operating the chair is fatiguing. But many modern wheelchairs are extremely light and fold up easily, making them highly portable. Motorized chairs are a great help to many people with more advanced MS. They are not usually meant for all-day sitting, though, and you'll likely need a manual wheelchair as well. Many people feel overjoyed at the enhanced mobility a motorized wheelchair or scooter provides. They are able to again "walk" around the mall, or go for rides to the park, and they are generally less fatigued. The psychological and practical benefits are considerable and justify the significant cost of a motorized vehicle.

The key reason for choosing a chair or scooter is improving your independence. Ask a physiotherapist or occupational therapist to help you pick the right one. The wiser your choice, the more mobile you will be.

Unsteadiness and Dizziness

Whether we are standing, sitting or lying down, we need balance. The cerebellum, in the brain, is the main center for balance, but the eyes, ears and spinal cord connections to the nerves to the arms and legs also play a role. MS may cause balance to worsen, particularly if the cerebellum (or connections to and from it) is affected. Unfortunately, no effective medications to improve balance are available. If a deterioration in balance is due to a relapse in MS, however, treatment with steroids sometimes works.

An unproven technique to improve balance is *vestibular stimulation*. The theory is that stimulating the balance centers in the brain somehow allows them to function more normally. The physiotherapist challenges your sense of balance by rocking, swinging or spinning you in different ways.

Another as yet unproven therapy is *computerized balance stimulation*. For this, you stand on a platform connected, through a computer, to a video screen. Movements of your feet produce changes on the screen. Through biofeedback, the theory says, you learn to achieve better balance.

Both vestibular stimulation and computerized balance stimulation should be considered research efforts in progress; neither is yet standard therapy.

Sometimes MS that involves the brainstem causes dizziness or vertigo (a spinning sensation). Frequently no treatment works well for the dizziness. A number of medications may help control vertigo, including *dimenhydrinate, prochlorperazine* and *ondansetron*. Their most frequent side effect is sedation, but they are quite helpful and should be used if the vertigo is sufficiently annoying, which it usually is.

Physical therapists can teach you exercises that will effectively control vertigo that is made worse by changes in head position. The therapist first determines which positions of the head worsen the vertigo. Therapy consists of holding the head in these positions for as long as possible. If you do this successfully, you will develop some tolerance and achieve greater comfort. The trouble is that vertigo in MS is rarely clearly positional in nature. Attacks recur regardless of head position.

Nausea and vomiting often accompany severe vertigo. Taking medications by mouth may not be possible, but physicians can inject antinausea drugs (the same ones used for vertigo). If the vertigo is part of a general flare-up of MS, treatment with steroids may be necessary, as in the case of all relapses.

Shaking, or Tremors

Tremors are to-and-fro movements of the extremities or, occasionally, the head and neck. They may be minimal, moderate or severe. Some occur at rest; others only happen during purposeful movements. Some are fast and some are slow. These factors determine how physicians treat MS-related tremors. Some respond quite well to treatment; others are extremely difficult to treat, and quite disabling. Maximizing function is the goal in treating the tremors.

Physiological Tremor

From time to time probably all of us have noticed a fine shaking when our arms are outstretched. It is what causes a cup of coffee to shake in our hands as we bring it to our lips. This type of tremor is in no way specific to MS. It responds well to medications called beta blockers, such as *propranolol*. A few people develop low blood pressure taking beta blockers, but the drugs are quite safe, although they can worsen asthma and should not be used by people with congestive heart failure. Physiological tremor may increase with anxiety or fatigue.

Rest Tremor

Some medications, particularly certain tranquilizers, can cause a tremor when a person is at rest. Adjusting the dosage or using counteracting drugs helps.

Cerebellar Tremor

Unfortunately, the most common tremor in MS, and the most difficult to treat, results from demyelination in the area of the cerebellum, the part of the brain responsible for balance and for coordinating muscle movement. Typically, demyelination in the cerebellum causes a major tremor called *intention tremor*. It can be severe, and occurs with purposeful movements of the arms or legs. For example, when the person tries to bring a spoon to the mouth, the arm shakes at right angles to the intended direction of the spoon. In some cases the arm shakes so badly that it has to be restrained, and purposeful movement of the limb is impossible. When the limb is at rest, however, there is little or no tremor.

Unfortunately, no drug consistently and significantly treats this disabling symptom, although medical textbooks mention tranquilizers, beta blockers, antiseizure drugs such as *primidone*, even water pills such as *acetazolamide*, or *isoniazid*, a drug used to treat tuberculosis. New medications are being tried, but whether they work is uncertain.

Sometimes physicians attempt to manage cerebellar tremor with non-drug treatments:

- *Immobilization* involves placing a brace across the joint so that the joint is fixed in one position. This lessens the severity of the tremor by reducing random movement. Bracing helps most in the ankle and foot because it provides a stable base for standing and walking. Occasionally, an arm and hand are braced so someone can write, eat or knit.
- *Weighting* also increases control over erratic limb movements. It reduces tremor and possibly provides greater sensory feedback to the brain. Either the limb itself is weighted—by wrapping a weight around the wrist, for example—or the object being used—such as a utensil, pen or pencil, cane or walker—is made heavier.

Although these techniques reduce the tremors themselves, the goal is to teach you to compensate for the tremors by providing as much stability for your limbs as possible. Nonskid, easy-to-grasp, stable equipment and/or assistive devices will help with eating, dressing, cooking and homemaking. Examples include walkers with lockable brakes and bathrooms with grip bars. An occupational therapist will have lots of suggestions.

Tremors of the head, neck and upper torso are hard to treat. Stabilizing the neck with a brace may help.

Tremors of the lips, tongue or jaw may affect speech by interfering with the breath control needed for phrasing and loudness; they may also affect the person's ability to make sounds. Speech therapy teaches you to increase your ability to communicate efficiently. It may involve learning to change the rate of speaking or the phrasing of sentences.

None of these techniques completely eliminates the problems associated with tremor. In fact, for some people with MS, tremor is the most disabling symptom. In certain cases, physicians consider surgery to areas deep in the brain that affect tremor. But brain surgery is not without significant risk. It is done only rarely, and to date the results have not been especially encouraging in MS, as the benefits tend to be temporary, at best.

Swallowing Problems

Swallowing problems are not uncommon in MS, particularly in more advanced cases. The medical term for difficulty in swallowing is *dysphagia*. Swallowing passes food from the mouth into the throat, past the breathing passage and down the esophagus to the stomach. Food may stick in the throat, blocking the air passage, or travel sluggishly down the esophagus, causing coughing, sputtering and anxiety; or, even more dangerously, it may go down the breathing passage and on toward the lungs. People who are with you when you eat should be trained in how to deal with a choking emergency.

Symptoms of swallowing problems include gurgling, sounds of congestion, spitting or coughing after meals, weight loss, pneumonia, sore throat, choking, a weak voice or an inability to "get the food down." Always take swallowing difficulties seriously and have them properly investigated.

After a neurological examination to assess the movement of the muscles in the mouth and throat, the best way to evaluate swallowing problems is to X-ray the mouth and throat as the person swallows. This allows the radiologist and speech pathologist (who also helps to assess and manage swallowing difficulties) to see exactly where the problem lies.

The goal of treatment is to improve nutrition while making swallowing safe. Modifying food textures may help, since some foods are swallowed more easily than others. For example, sometimes a thickening agent or a gelatin must be added. Nuts need to be limited because they stick in the throat and may be irritating. Semisolid food is the easiest to swallow. Food that is warm or cold may help stimulate a swallow reflex. Other maneuvers include making sure you tilt your head back during eating, alternating solids and liquids so that food doesn't stick in the throat, and eating more frequent but smaller-volume meals. In more difficult cases food may need to be puréed. If none of these techniques is effective, a feeding tube can be inserted into the stomach through the nose, or directly into the stomach, surgically, to maintain adequate nutrition.

Swollen Ankles

People with MS whose legs are weak sometimes develop swollen ankles and calves. This is due to an accumulation of fluid from either veins or lymphatic channels. (Veins bring blood back to the heart, and lymphatics carry protein-rich lymphatic fluid to the heart.) Normally the action of the leg muscles pumps this fluid back toward the heart. When movement is impaired, gravity causes the fluid to pool in the ankles and feet.

Treatment is relatively simple, and consists of elevating the feet so they are higher than the hips for periods of time during the day and throughout the night, so that gravity moves the fluid back toward the trunk. Support stockings help to keep the lymph fluid within its normal channels, but they must fit properly to avoid pinching the leg muscles. Water pills (diuretics) are not usually recommended for this type of swelling because they don't work well or, if they do, the fluid quickly returns, even when you continue on the medication.

Two serious conditions also cause swelling of the ankles, and for this reason your physician should assess the problem when it occurs. Fluid pooling in the ankles may indicate that the heart is not functioning properly. In this case other symptoms such as shortness of breath, coughing and a general feeling of weakness are also usually present. Swelling in one leg, together with redness and pain, may mean you have a deep venous thrombosis (blood clot in a vein). This condition is potentially fatal, and requires immediate investigation and treatment with blood thinners.

Usually, however, swelling of the ankles is a benign symptom in MS, more a nuisance than a sign of a major problem.

Weight Gain

Weight gain may become a problem in MS, especially if your mobility decreases but the amount you eat remains the same. Weight gain also results from steroid or antidepressant use. Excessive weight makes general movement harder, and makes actions such as changing position more difficult than necessary.

To control your weight, strive to achieve a balance between calories, exercise and rest. This may mean eating smaller meals. Many people find that having small but frequent meals lowers their overall caloric intake and is even more satisfying than eating large meals.

Dietary Guidelines

No diet has ever been proven to modify the course of MS. However, one school of thought holds that a diet low in saturated fats is beneficial—specifically, a diet high in monounsaturated and polyunsaturated fats such as those found in olive oil and fish oil.

The fish-oil hypothesis was tested in the 1970s in England. A large group of people with MS was assembled and divided into two. One half was given a fish-oil supplement and the other was not. After several years of observation, researchers found no significant difference between the two, although there was a trend in favor of the fish-oil group.

Another diet theory holds that MS is caused by a kind of intolerance to "new" foods such as wheat and dairy products. Proponents of this diet recommend eliminating these foods, as in the diet used to treat celiac disease (a bowel disorder). Speak to a dietitian if you want the details of this diet.

Other diet studies have been so poorly designed and carried out that they are inconclusive. The truth is that we still don't know whether diet has something to do with people getting MS, or with the way the disease progresses.

It is easy to see how the notion that diet is important would take hold. MS is inherently variable, with relapses and remissions once or twice a year, followed by periods of recovery. If people with MS go on a special diet just as they start to improve, they are likely to attribute their improvement to the diet when in fact they would have improved anyway.

What kind of diet should you follow? A low-fat diet is recommended. It almost certainly won't harm you. It may help your MS. And if it doesn't, it will at least reduce your risk of heart disease and certain kinds of cancer. So eat your vegetables and fruits and avoid too many fatty foods. A nutritionist can help you here. I cannot routinely recommend more demanding diets, such as the celiac diet, until there is more evidence from clinical trials.

Alcohol

Unless it's forbidden for other reasons, an occasional social drink will do no harm. If you have fatigue, balance or bladder symptoms, liquor may increase them, and it may be wise to limit your consumption. On the other hand, you may find that a drink helps you relax when anxiety or tension worsens your symptoms. Moderation—meaning no more than one or two drinks per day—is the key. Be sure to check with your doctor first, though, if you're taking any medication.

Pressure Sores

Occasionally, people with advanced multiple sclerosis develop pressure sores (also called bedsores)—breaks in the skin, like red craters, which result from too much pressure. Most people who develop them are immobilized or move only minimally over long periods of time. They have decreased sensation in their skin and do not feel the discomfort that would normally tell them that they have been in one position for too long. Pressure sores most commonly occur on the buttocks and other places in constant contact with a bed or wheelchair. They frequently appear with little or no pain, and continue to enlarge, gradually expanding into the underlying muscle. Other factors that contribute to their development are inadequate nutrition, certain medications, stool or urine incontinence and a lack of education about prevention.

The key to managing pressure sores is to prevent them in the first place.

- Change position frequently to transfer weight off contact areas, but be careful not to create friction in the process. You may need someone to help you do this.
- Use proper equipment—foam pillows, air mattresses, water mattresses, gels—to spread body weight over larger areas.
- Put foam rubber pads and sheepskins under pressure points such as the sacrum (base of the spinal column) and heels to help spread the pressure.
- Examine the skin frequently for areas of redness and broken skin.

If an ulcer develops, see a physician right away. Do not apply pressure to the area. Wash the wound with a solution of hydrogen peroxide or saline, both available from your drugstore, but keep the surrounding skin dry. Many different dressings (bandages) are available. If the pressure sore is minor, covering it with "artificial skin" (polyurethane film dressing) will keep it from becoming infected and allow it to heal. Sometimes, placing a 100-watt lamp 18 to 24 inches (45 to 60 cm) from the wound for 10 minutes several times a day helps. An alternating pressure mattress, a specialized bed that protects all skin surfaces by automatically shifting pressures to different parts of the body, can help prevent or treat pressure sores.

Larger pressure sores require ongoing attention from a physician, usually a plastic surgeon, and a nurse, for frequent cleaning of the wound, and other treatment. The process is lengthy but usually successful.

Numbness

Numbness is one of the most common complaints in MS. It is more annoying than disabling, except when it interferes with motor coordination of the limbs. It occurs when the nerves that transmit feeling do not conduct information properly.

There is no medication to reduce numbness, but when the numbness happens as part of a relapse, steroids decrease the intensity of the relapse and hasten recovery. Steroids are not often used if numbness is the only symptom of a relapse, but they can be tried if the numbness causes clumsiness. If the numbness is associated with pain or uncomfortable tingling, amitriptyline or *gabapentin* may help (see "Pain" in this chapter).

The best way to deal with numbness is to ignore it, if possible. Its presence does not necessarily imply that the disease is getting worse.

Sexuality Problems

Sexual response depends on a sequence of reflexes involving neural transmissions stimulated by a wide variety of sensations. Electrical signals from the brain travel to the genitals via the spinal cord through nerves (*nervi erigentes*) that exit near the bottom of the spinal cord, near the bowel and bladder reflex centers. The nerve pathways between the brain and genitals are long and complex, and any problem in the nerves can cause short circuits in the system, producing sexual dysfunction. It is not surprising, therefore, that sexual difficulties often arise in people with MS.

Over 90 percent of men with MS and 70 percent of women report negative changes in their sex life after the onset of the disease. Women report impaired genital sensation, diminished orgasmic response and loss of interest; they may also be bothered by intense itching, diminished vaginal lubrication, weak vaginal muscles and a reflexive pulling together of the legs (called *adductor spasms*) during intercourse. Men most frequently report impaired genital sensation, decreased sex drive, difficulty in achieving an erection and delayed ejaculation or decreased force of ejaculation. Both men and women report negative effects on self-esteem.

If You're a Woman
To avoid bowel/bladder and catheter problems during intercourse, reduce fluids about two hours before sexual activity and empty the bladder before lovemaking. Be prepared in case an accident occurs despite precautions, and remember that it is not a catastrophe. A vaginal lubricant such as KY Jelly may be necessary.

Minimize leg spasms by timing an antispasticity medication so that its effect is at a peak during sexual activity. Have intercourse in a side position with bent knees, or use pillows for support if "legs together" spasms are a problem. Try a vibrator; it sometimes compensates for the loss of deep pressure sense in MS that impairs vaginal sensation. A variety of different vibrators are available. *Sildenafil* (Viagra) does not appear to work in women, whether or not they have MS.

If You're a Man
Much can be done to improve impaired erections. Typically, seeing a urologist is the first step.

Clinical studies suggest that sildenafil (Viagra) and its chemical cousins, Levitra and Cialis, can help many men with MS who are having problems with impotence. These are the drugs I recommend first. Side effects can include headache and, in men who already have heart disease, heart problems.

Injection medications, such as *papaverine* and *alprostadil*, go into the shaft of the penis or into the tip of the urethra just prior to intercourse. Although they provide a natural erection, you must be able to overcome any fear of injecting medication into the penis. In isolated instances, repeated injections have caused scarring of the penis. Occasionally, an erection that won't go away (priapism) occurs with injections. This painful side effect can be treated medically in an emergency department.

Another approach to impotence is to implant a surgical prosthesis in the penis. It may be a rigid noninflatable rod prosthesis or a semirigid inflatable device.

Another method that does not call for an injection is the penile vacuum device. A tube is placed over the penis, with a rubber band around the top of the tube. A pump removes the air from the tube, creating a vacuum that draws blood into the penis to produce an erection. After the erection is achieved, you slide the rubber band under the base of the penis and remove the tube. The rubber band can safely maintain a firm erection for up to 30 minutes. Although the erection is not as firm as a normal or a drug-induced one, it is quite functional. As yet, there is no drug to help men ejaculate.

A diagnosis of MS can have negative effects on someone's self-image. People who have visible disability commonly feel less attractive sexually, and are concerned about obstacles such as braces, wheelchairs and catheters. The key is to become comfortable with your body, a goal that requires time, patience and commitment, and is difficult given our "beauty-oriented" modern culture with its relentless emphasis on youthful physical perfection.

Look for your positive qualities as a person, and put effort into feeling good about yourself by taking care of your body through exercise, diet and dress. Feeling good about yourself as a person helps beat the myth that you must have a "perfect body" to be sexy.

In relationships, deal with feelings openly and honestly. Let your partner know what feels good and what does not; experiment with sexual positions and create alternative ways to give and receive pleasure. Sex should not be goal oriented, with intercourse and orgasm the only focus. Many people get great physical and psychological satisfaction from foreplay. One way to decrease or eliminate pressures and high expectations is to rename such activities "sex play" and recognize that they have value in themselves. Sexual expression may be directed to parts of the body other than the genitals, and may include cuddling, caressing, massage or other forms of touch; it may involve experimenting with oral sex, masturbation, vibrators and other devices. Many people require "permission" from their partners to become less inhibited in their imagination, and in expressing their sexuality. Don't be afraid to ask.

You and your partner need to deal with emotions such as anxiety, guilt, anger, depression and denial. As a couple, you should also be aware that sometimes these painful feelings do not lessen or disappear, despite communication and support. You may need to seek professional help to deal with persistent negative feelings, or use helpful medications such as antidepressants.

While doctors have made great strides in diagnosing sexual difficulties and providing alternative treatments, much remains to be done, particularly in improving the sexual responsiveness of women whose excitation and orgasm are defective because of MS-impaired sensation or reflexes. The key remains good communication between you and your partner, and between you and your health care team. In some cases, though not all, a focused, open-minded approach to sexual problems will result in a satisfying sex life. The ability to be honest and frank with your partner is the single most important element in creating intimacy and enhancing your sex life.

Alternative Therapies

People are turning to alternative medicine in greater numbers every year. This is not because modern medicine is less effective than in the past. On the contrary, there are more treatments now than ever. But we have a greater expectation of good health nowadays. To some extent, this rising expectation is nurtured by stories in the media, which often exaggerate the latest medical advance. If conventional medicine cannot supply the expected cure, people tend to look elsewhere.

If you wanted to design a disease that is a charlatan's dream, you could not do better than MS. It is a chronic illness with long periods of remission and occasional relapses. The cause is unknown and the treatment is far from satisfactory. Therefore, if you happen to give somebody an alternative therapy just as the disease goes into remission, he or she will attribute the recovery to that treatment. If the treatment goes badly, you can blame the person for not using enough or the right type of your potion or diet, and proceed to the next level of "treatment." Since the cause of the disease is unknown, even the most ludicrous theory can be given a surface plausibility by the glib.

The alternative therapies discussed below are "non-establishment" in the sense that they are not generally prescribed by physicians, due to a lack of scientific evidence in favor of their use. Some of these therapies have never been properly evaluated for either effectiveness or safety in appropriately designed long-term randomized controlled trials. However, that does not necessarily mean that they are not effective, or not safe.

Every week, the newspapers bring us reports of new miracle "cures" or "treatments" for MS. People frequently ask their physicians about this or that alternative therapy, particularly nutritional and vitamin-type supplements. As individuals living in a free society, they have a perfect right to undertake any legal treatment they wish. But it is obviously unwise to experiment with any unproven therapies that carry significant health risks.

There are some aspects of alternative therapies that are undoubtedly beneficial. For example, with any form of therapy there is a *placebo effect*. That is, the very fact of having a treatment—even if the treatment is completely inactive—improves symptoms, at least temporarily, in about one-quarter to one-third of patients. So if someone reports symptomatic improvements from a safe treatment that sounds useless, the correct response is "Fine."

Alternative therapies may give someone a positive outlook and some optimism about the future. The practitioner may spend time with the patient, giving sympathy, reassurance and good advice. There may even be genuine therapeutic action from an alternative therapy.

On the negative side, any treatment carries the potential of harm. Seemingly innocent herbs can cause all sorts of medical problems. Acupuncture done in the wrong place can cause a pneumothorax (punctured lung). Non-sterile needles carry the risk of hepatitis or AIDS. In addition, someone may abandon conventional therapy and rely solely on alternative therapies, missing out on the proven benefits of established medicine. Moreover, people who feel great optimism at the beginning of an alternative therapy may be deeply depressed if the condition worsens despite the therapy. As well, alternative therapies can be costly—particularly for MS patients, who usually have limited financial resources.

In short: discuss alternative therapies with your physician. If you decide to proceed, avoid anything that seems unsafe, and compare the costs of the treatment with its potential benefits.

Acupuncture

This is an ancient Chinese method of treatment introduced to the West by a 17th-century Dutch physician. In 1923 the British medical journal *The Lancet* reported its successful use in treating rheumatism. Acupuncture is based on the belief that there is a balance in the body between two universal forces or principles known as *yin* and *yang*, and that there are 14 meridians extending like trunk roads over the body, each linking acupuncture points. In the treatment, fine needles are inserted into the relevant points and are stimulated by twisting with the fingers or by means of a lead clipped to the needle which is then stimulated by an electro-acupuncture device. There is a slight prick when the needle goes in, and stimulation of the needle produces a heavy numbness or tingling sensation.

It is possible that this stimulation produces activity in certain rapidly acting pain fibers, resulting in the release of endorphins, the body's natural painkillers. Acupuncture therapy may also promote the release of steroids, which can have a beneficial effect on many painful conditions. Thus acupuncture may be useful in treating pain associated with multiple sclerosis. It does not alter the progression of the disease.

Aromatherapy
This treatment consists of using highly concentrated scented plant oils, either massaged onto the body or inhaled or added to a hot bath (but remember that hot baths can worsen MS symptoms). Aromatherapy may help in relaxation. It has no other specific use in multiple sclerosis.

Chiropractic
A charismatic healer named Daniel Palmer started this form of treatment, based on physical manipulation, in 1895. It may be useful in relieving back pain but has no specific role in multiple sclerosis management. No scientific study has ever proved that spinal manipulation worsens the prognosis of people with MS, but no study has ever shown that it helps. Neck manipulation may be unsafe because it may irritate the spinal cord or cause other neurological damage such as strokes. For these reasons I never recommend neck manipulation for people with MS.

Cold Immersion
Exposure to heat, as in hot weather or a hot bath, can produce dramatic temporary worsening of neurological symptoms. Cooling tends to have the opposite effect. Some patients report much-improved function after cooling in a swimming pool. Cooling treatments such as a cool bath or swim are safe, inexpensive and harmless. They are recommended for people whose symptoms are particularly temperature-sensitive. Expensive cooling vests are not usually necessary.

Dietary Supplements

Vitamins are the first supplement most patients ask me about. A multivitamin is recommended, although trials of MS patients have not produced any evidence to support their use. Because inadequate vitamin D_3 may be associated with the risk of MS, I suggest a daily vitamin D_3 supplement of 2,000 to 4,000 MIU. (MIU stands for "million International Units.") Although there is no proof that this helps, it is unlikely to do any harm.

Many people ask about dietary supplements of polyunsaturated fats such as linoleic acid, sunflower seed oil, safflower seed oil or evening primrose oil. The theory is that these substances can be used by the body to synthesize other fatty acids that are important constituents of myelin in the CNS. However, no consistent abnormalities of these unsaturated fatty acids have been identified in MS patients.

Several studies have been performed using polyunsaturated fatty acids including sunflower seed oil, evening primrose oil and safflower seed oil. One study reported some reduction in frequency of relapses, whereas another reported a reduction in the severity of attacks but no change in frequency and the third failed to find any favorable effect. People with minimal disability at the beginning of the trial appeared to do best.

The good thing about using polyunsaturated fatty acids is that no significant toxic effects have been reported. Some people don't like the taste of the pure oil and tolerate emulsions, spreads or capsules better. Occasionally, people develop diarrhea from these oils. The long-term effects of high polyunsaturated fatty acid intake are unknown, but at least the cost of these oils is relatively modest.

In all, the treatment may have some benefits but so far the evidence is contradictory. On the other hand, there seems to be no strong reason against trying it, if you wish to do so.

The same applies to fatty acids of fish oil. A large multi-center double-blind trial of the effect of dietary supplementation with various fatty acids of fish oil was performed in Great Britain. (In a double-blind trial, neither the subjects nor the doctors know what substance is being administered.) There was a trend in favor of the treatment but it did not reach statistical significance, and many people did not like the fishy taste associated with large doses of the oil.

Herbal Medicines

Herbal medicines have been around for thousands of years, and some have been purified, scientifically verified and accepted as medical treatments. It has been estimated that 50 percent of medications prescribed by family physicians are plant-based. However, no herbal therapies are of proven benefit in the treatment of MS. Also, in conventional medicine the active ingredient is isolated, purified and served up in exact doses. With herbal medicines, you can never be certain of the exact dose you are getting, and the product may contain additional substances that are useless or even dangerous.

Homeopathy

Homeopathy was developed by a German physician who believed that naturally occurring substances producing symptoms *resembling* those of an ailment could, if greatly diluted, be used to treat the ailment itself. Plant and mineral substances are most widely used. They are soaked in alcohol and then vastly diluted. There are no homeopathic treatments of proven use in the treatment of MS, and the principles of homeopathy have not been confirmed in scientific trials.

In addition to the lack of scientific evidence for the efficacy of homeopathic treatments, there is a commonsense objection as well. There is no reason why producing the symptoms of an illness should help to treat it. In addition, the preparations are so dilute that they seem unlikely to do much of anything, positive or negative.

Injections of Venom

Snake Venom

The idea of using snake venom in MS treatment developed when a person who worked with snakes was bitten. He suffered various neurological symptoms, some of which suggested stimulation of the nervous system. Snake venom has also been looked at as a treatment for arthritis, lupus, herpes infections, muscular dystrophy, Parkinson's disease, myasthenia gravis and amyotrophic lateral sclerosis.

The treatment consists of injections of the venom. There are several different preparations available in different countries. Pain and swelling occur at the injection site, although these tend to diminish as the injections are repeated over days to weeks. One bad allergic reaction has been reported. Given the absence of an objective controlled study looking at the use of snake venoms, the lack of a standardized preparation of known composition and proven safety and the possibility of a life-threatening allergic reaction, this treatment is not recommended.

Bee Venom

Bee venom therapy involves either injecting extracts of the venom or having bees sting the patient once or several times per day. The treatment is quite painful, and is typically used by people with moderate to severe disability. Some report temporarily increased energy, strength and walking ability. The potential for serious and even life-threatening allergic reactions is very real. Anaphylaxis (allergic shock) can occur in anyone who undertakes this therapy. Epinephrine (adrenaline) must be at hand in case of an allergic reaction, and the person must know how to use it. If epinephrine is required, medical help must also be sought immediately, in case the reaction proves to be severe.

Bee venom has been shown not to be effective in animals with an MS-like disease. Currently, bee venom therapy is being examined in a small safety trial of patients with progressive multiple sclerosis. We do not know yet if this treatment is effective and safe enough for routine clinical use. It is certainly inexpensive and readily available, but it seems unlikely to have any significant long-term benefit. Patients of mine who try this painful treatment report, at best, an increase in energy level that soon wears off. Inevitably, they soon abandon the injections.

Massage

Massage may be useful in the treatment of MS, for relief of spasticity and pain. A qualified massage therapist may be very helpful. Massage should be used as part of an overall rehabilitation regime, and massage techniques that are particularly painful should be avoided.

Meditation

The general aim of meditation is to achieve a tranquil state of mind. The principles have been around for thousands of years. The relaxation produced in association with meditation is certainly harmless, and may well assist you in coping with the physical and psychological burdens of MS. See also "Yoga," below.

Reflexology

Reflexologists use charts of the feet marked off in zones to represent all parts of the body. Massage of the appropriate zone is supposed to clear energy channels, allowing the body to heal. The assumptions of this theory appear dubious, but foot massage may certainly assist in producing relaxation.

Tai Chi

Tai chi is a pattern of flowing movements combined with relaxation and meditation techniques, developed in China in the eleventh century. Each individual movement is fairly easy but requires a degree of balance, flexibility and relaxation. The movements are exact and demand a great deal of concentration. Some of the advantages of tai chi are that people of any age can participate—even from wheelchairs—and the training is inexpensive. This is certainly a harmless treatment, and may help improve muscle flexibility as well as mental well-being.

Yoga

Yoga is a meditation and exercise technique. There are different forms; hatha yoga, for instance, concentrates on postures, while raja yoga focuses on mental control. The benefits of yoga include flexibility, relaxation and some increase in muscle strength.

SIX

Treating the Disease: Present and Future

The 1990s will be remembered, by people with MS, as the decade in which disease-modifying treatments became available. By this we mean that physicians can now treat the underlying condition rather than just the symptoms. Let's take an infected tooth as an example. A painkiller relieves the pain (symptom); antibiotics and/or dental surgery constitute the disease-modifying treatment that fixes the problem. The treatments discussed in Chapter Five alleviate MS symptoms. However, none halts or slows the underlying MS. Naturally, symptom therapies have their place, but the real goal with any disease is to find a treatment that eliminates the disease or, at the very least, slows down its progress.

Up until 1993, we had no disease-modifying therapies for MS. Despite the huge number of treatments proposed by one or another medical or nonmedical authority over the years, none had survived the rigors of scientific trials. In 1993, the results of a large clinical trial conducted throughout North America over several years showed that treatment with *interferon beta 1b* (Betaseron) reduced the number of MS attacks by about a third over a three-year period. In large-scale studies published since

1993, three other drugs have shown an effect in reducing the number of attacks. Two involve *interferon beta 1a* (Avonex and Rebif) and the other involves a small protein fragment known as *glatiramer acetate* (Copaxone). So far, these drugs have shown definite success with relapsing-remitting MS only.

Interferon Beta in Relapsing-Remitting MS

Interferon beta 1a and interferon beta 1b are proteins that are very similar to each other; the former is identical to human interferon beta, whereas the latter is slightly different. Interferon beta is normally produced by white blood cells. It modifies the normal activity of the immune system, which attacks the central nervous system in MS. It has a number of different effects, some of which are not very well understood, but in general it seems to decrease immune activity and, among other things, block white blood cells (lymphocytes)—the infantry in the immune-system army—from entering the brain. We know that the lymphocytes migrate through blood vessels into the brain across what is called the *blood-brain barrier*, a tissue barrier that allows some substances, but not all, to migrate from the bloodstream into the brain itself. Interferons beta 1b and beta 1a act as "sealants" to inhibit this migration. It's like injecting a sealant into a flat tire to plug a leak.

Interferon Beta 1b (Betaseron)

In the 1993 study, treatment with interferon beta 1b resulted in fewer relapses, milder relapses when they did occur and fewer hospitalizations for relapses. Significantly, MRI scans showed that the amount of disease in the brain in people treated with the drug was less than in those treated with a placebo. In other words, the drug appeared to have a physical effect on what was going on in the brain. On the basis of its effects on relapses and MRI scans, the drug was approved in North America and Europe as the first disease-modifying treatment for relapsing-remitting MS.

Another, smaller study in the United States showed that interferon beta 1b may slow the deterioration in cognitive function—for example, memory—that happens in MS over time.

The medication is injected subcutaneously (under the skin) every two days. Self-injection may make you squeamish, but it's simple to learn, and learning takes no more than an hour or two in the vast majority of cases. The injections are done in the thighs, buttocks or abdomen, areas typically rich in fat, to minimize pain and skin reaction. If you are one of a small minority of people with a needle phobia, a nurse or a family physician can give you the injections.

Side Effects

Interferon beta 1b has some side effects. Injection-site reactions are common. These include redness, bruising and pain, shrinkage of tissue at the site and necrosis, meaning a breakdown of the skin with secondary infection. There seem to be fewer local skin reactions when injections are done in the buttocks. Injecting into the arms appears to be especially painful. Many people find it easiest to inject into the abdomen. Remember never to inject in the same place repeatedly, and to inject deep enough under the skin to minimize skin reactions.

More generalized side effects can also occur. The most important is a flulike reaction that begins within 24 hours of the injection and can last one to three days, or occasionally even longer. During this period you feel as if you have the flu, with headache, fatigue, chills, sore muscles and fever. About 60 percent of all people experience at least some of these symptoms. They can be minimized by taking acetaminophen or ibuprofen one hour before the injection and every six to twelve hours thereafter for a day or two, as necessary. These symptoms are particularly a problem just after you start the therapy, and in most cases disappear within two or three months if not before.

Taking the drug at bedtime may enable you to sleep through these symptoms. The flulike symptoms are more common in women than in men receiving the same dose of medication, suggesting that they are related to body weight. If the flulike side effects are intolerable, start the drug at half the recommended dose for the first two to four weeks and slowly increase it.

Other side effects are rare. Some people report an increase in spasticity. Very rarely, minor abnormalities show up in liver function tests, and in the number of white blood cells. However, these usually resolve on their own. The drug seems safe to use with other medications.

Some 30 to 40 percent of people treated develop antibodies (proteins in their blood) over time. Whether or not these antibodies affect the drug's effectiveness is unclear, and is a matter of great controversy. Ask your neurologist for the latest information on this complex subject.

The drug starts to work after two months of treatment. Because it is associated with side effects during those two months, it is not uncommon for people to feel worse right after starting therapy, or for their MS symptoms to worsen before gradually stabilizing. Many people feel worse the day after an injection, then better the following day. Therapies for MS symptoms can be used at the same time as interferon beta 1b.

Who Should Get Interferon Beta 1b?

Only people with confirmed MS (see Chapter Four) should receive this treatment, and only if they have active relapsing-remitting MS, which means in general about two significant attacks in the previous few years. Your neurologist can supply you with further details.

The drug is probably not appropriate for people with very mild relapsing-remitting disease—only one or two sensory attacks over many years—as it is unlikely that the treatment will improve what is already quite a mild situation.

As well, you should not use this medication if:

- you are allergic to any component of the drug;
- you are suffering from severe depression;
- you are pregnant, nursing or trying to become pregnant.

When Should You Stop the Drug?

People who respond well to interferon beta 1b—who have fewer relapses and tolerate the drug without significant persistent side effects—should continue the therapy for three years or more. Those who do not have a good response—who have intolerable side effects, no decrease in relapses requiring steroid treatment or a clear increase in disability over the course of a year's treatment—should probably discontinue the drug. Whether or not to stop using the drug should be an individual decision made after discussion with your neurologist. Every case is different.

Interferon Beta 1a (Avonex, Rebif)

The first major report on the effectiveness of interferon beta 1a appeared in 1996. Another report, on a second large study, came out in 1998. The drug was studied in similar but not identical populations of people with relapsing-remitting multiple sclerosis. In both studies, the relapses appeared to decrease by about a third. The drug also appeared to slow the development of disability. Like interferon beta 1b, interferon beta 1a seemed to have a beneficial effect on the amount of disease observed in the brain on MRI scan.

Although they are made by different companies, the two drugs are chemically identical. Perhaps the most important distinguishing feature between the drugs is that Avonex is taken only once a week, whereas Rebif is taken three times a week. Avonex is injected into the muscle, whereas Rebif is injected just under the skin. You can teach yourself to do either type of injection, although learning to inject into muscle is a little more challenging. Injecting once a week is certainly more convenient than injecting every two days. In addition, because you inject more deeply into muscle than you do subcutaneously, local skin reactions are insignificant with Avonex. Whether injecting once a week gives as much benefit as injecting every two days is still controversial.

Which is the best way to take interferon beta 1a? In a head-to-head study of Avonex and Rebif in 2002, Rebif was associated with a higher chance of remaining relapse-free over 12 months and having fewer new lesions appearing on MRI scans. However, Rebif was also associated with more skin reactions, liver-enzyme changes and *neutralizing antibodies*. The latter are proteins that the body produces in response to the interferon. Over time, neutralizing antibodies can negate the beneficial effects of the interferon.

Side Effects
Side effects include the flulike symptoms commonly seen with interferon beta 1b. The timing of the injection (usually before bed), side effects and pretreatment with acetaminophen or ibuprofen are the same as with interferon beta 1b.

Who Should Get Interferon Beta 1a?
The criteria and contraindications are similar to those for interferon beta 1b, but people treated with 1a (particularly Avonex) are much less likely to develop antibodies than people receiving 1b. For people with only one attack, Avonex is most effective. Which drug is best suited to you is a decision for you to make after detailed consultation with your neurologist.

Glatiramer Acetate (Copaxone)

In 1995, the results of a study of glatiramer acetate in the treatment of relapsing-remitting MS were published. Glatiramer acetate—the brand name is Copaxone—is a small fragment of a protein that resembles a protein in myelin. Exactly how it works is unclear, but one theory is that it turns off the unwanted activity of the immune system. We don't know if it "seals" the blood-brain barrier, but it does seem to decrease the lymphocytes' attack on the myelin. Whether it can be used along with interferon beta 1b and 1a remains to be determined, although a preliminary study presented in 2002 suggests that the combination of Avonex and Copaxone is safe.

This drug, too, appears to decrease relapses by about a third. In the original study, MRIs of people who had been treated with the drug were not systematically examined, so there was a subsequent study on whether the drug slows disease in the brain. The results showed a modest beneficial effect on brain MRIs, not as great as the benefits of interferon beta 1a or interferon beta 1b. However, the interferon's beneficial effects are more apparent in the MRI than in the way the person feels.

Glatiramer acetate, like interferon 1b, is injected subcutaneously, but daily rather than every two days or every week. Side effects are minimal. The skin at the injection site may redden. With this drug no flulike reaction occurs. Occasionally, people experience a brief episode (a few minutes) of breathlessness. We don't know what causes this unusual reaction. It goes away on its own and appears to be self-limiting.

Like interferon beta 1b and 1a, the drug is used to treat relapsing-remitting MS. It is not approved for the treatment of progressive MS. Also like interferon beta 1b and 1a, glatiramer acetate should not be used if you are allergic to any of its components, or if you are pregnant, trying to become pregnant or nursing.

Interferon beta 1b, interferon beta 1a and glatiramer acetate: a summary

The three disease-modifying drugs approved for the treatment of relapsing-remitting MS have many similarities:

- They reduce MS relapses by about a third.

- They all have beneficial effects on brain MRI results, to varying degrees.

- They do not reverse existing disability, but they may stabilize the disease, although this does not happen for everyone.

- They must be injected.

- Side effects are usually manageable and self-limiting. Glatiramer acetate has the least side effects.

- Their overall effectiveness is modest.

- They are very expensive and people using them almost invariably require financial assistance from either an insurance company or a government program.

- Because of their modest effectiveness, significant cost and side effects, it's up to you to decide whether you want to use them and, if so, which one. Discuss the issue with your neurologist and your family.

Remember the fraction "one-third." All four drugs reduce relapses by about this much, and slow down the worsening of the MS, but they do not stop it. The benefits vary from person to person. Some people have no significant attacks while on the drug, and feel they've improved; others go on much the same, with recurrent, perhaps milder attacks of neurological symptoms; some people even get worse. These drugs do not reverse preexisting neurological symptoms. Unfortunately, although this is stated over and over, many people take these medications expecting that their symptoms will go away. Finally, beware of testimonials in which people with MS say that all their problems improved with these drugs. Because MS is by nature a highly variable condition, any given person might have gotten better even without the treatment.

Treatment for Progressive MS

Unfortunately, the current treatment situation for people with secondary progressive MS is much less encouraging. If you have this form of the disease *without frequent relapses*, it is unlikely that interferon beta 1a or interferon beta 1b will help you. The studies done in this area have been a little confusing because they include people both with and without relapses. However, my interpretation of the data is that only the people with relapses tended to benefit, and then only marginally, with a significant tradeoff in side effects, inconvenience and cost.

It may help to recall the discussion in Chapter One about the role that inflammation and degeneration (premature wearing out) play in producing damage in MS. Think of the relapsing-remitting phase as the early inflammatory stage of the illness. This phase responds to anti-inflammatory drugs that suppress the immune system, such as interferon beta (and in certain cases chemotherapy drugs; see below).

In the progressive phase, however, degeneration is the main cause of damage, and anti-inflammatory drugs do not slow down degeneration. For this phase we need *neuron-nurturing agents*. A number of these drugs are being looked at but, so far, none has been convincingly shown to benefit people with MS (or any other neurological degenerative disease, for that matter).

Chemotherapy agents include azathioprine, cladribine, methotrexate, cyclophosphamide and mitoxantrone. Chemotherapy suppresses the immune system, which is believed to be overactive in the brains of people with MS. But because it suppresses the immune system throughout the whole body, it leaves the body vulnerable to other "invasions" such as bacterial or viral diseases. Other potential serious side effects include damage to the white blood cells, infertility and infections of the liver, as well as creation of a cancer. Treating MS with chemotherapy is a bit like swatting a fly with a baseball bat—it may or may not work, but "collateral damage" is a definite possibility. Although chemotherapy has not worked convincingly for slowly progressing MS, many neurologists try it in people whose disease is rapidly worsening, and has not responded to drugs such as interferon beta and Copaxone. It's generally used in lower doses than in cancer therapy to minimize the risk, and is considered a treatment of last resort.

Mitoxantrone is approved in the U.S. and Europe for rapidly worsening MS, but the exact benefit of the drug remains to be clarified. It can sometimes damage the heart, particularily if it is used in doses that are too high.

Natalizumab (Tysabri) was approved in the United States in November 2004 for the treatment of relapsing-remitting MS on the basis of very encouraging one-year results (see pages 112–13) before its studies were completed.

Future Treatments

In the future, we hope to have treatments that will not only slow the rate of relapses and the progression of MS but actually stop the disease. Eventually, we hope to be able to reverse the neurological symptoms already present. Research is ongoing at many levels. As of spring 2003, over 120 different clinical trials were underway throughout the world. This quantity of research gives us a lot of hope for the future.

Seeking the Fundamental Mechanisms of MS

Researchers are doing a lot of work on how and why the immune system decides to attack the myelin. This usually means examining the steps involved in immune regulation, and trying to understand how genes control the function of the immune system. Finally, neuroscientists are intensely interested in remyelination, a repair process that could restore function to damaged parts of the nervous system. They have obtained several promising results using dog models of demyelination and remyelination.

There is also a lot of other symptom research going on, including looking at new drugs for memory loss (aricept or donepezil), pain (cannabinoids), and depression in MS.

Research into Symptoms

Many people with MS urgently want a drug to reduce the weakness they experience. Potassium channel blockers are mildly effective. Unfortunately, they occasionally have side effects, including dizziness and seizures. Further research is being done to produce drugs that reverse or dramatically improve the weakness without causing damaging side effects.

Research into Disease-modifying Treatments

Scientists are exploring several strategies to further modify the course of MS, including the use of proteins called *monoclonal antibodies* to target fragments of T lymphocytes (called T-cell receptors), or other components of the immune system. Vaccinating people with MS with certain components of the immune system is also under examination. The idea is to trick the body into producing proteins (antibodies) that attack and neutralize those parts of the immune system that provoke the MS in the first place. Will they work? Who knows?

Another approach is to inject proteins (called *selective adhesion molecule inhibitors*) to block the migration of those trouble-making lymphocytes into the brain and spinal cord. One of these compounds, natalizumab, is completing phase III trials in late 2004. Preliminary results from the first year of the study are very encouraging and include a remarkable 66 percent reduction in the number of relapses and a 92 percent reduction in the number of enhancing brain lesions in the treated group. The drug was safe and well tolerated with only occasional side effects.

In light of these very positive findings, the FDA approved the drug for use in MS in November 2004, before the final two-year results of the study were available. The medication is given only once per month, through an injection into the vein. It is expected to be quite expensive.

Researchers are also exploring transplantation of myelin-forming cells. At this point the results are interesting but still preliminary. This therapy is a long way from becoming reality, and it may never work. For one thing, it's very difficult to get the transplanted cells to the precise location where they are needed. Also, even if the myelin repairs itself, the underlying axon is often damaged as well, and a myelin transplant does nothing to fix that. Nonetheless, safety trials in humans have started.

Although rare, bone marrow transplantation has been tried in particularly aggressive cases of MS. This therapy is of unproven benefit and carries signigicant risk.

Other therapies have also been looked at. Because of the rapidly changing nature of this field, the best way to get a handle on MS research is to contact your local multiple sclerosis society, and to keep an eye on the newspaper or television. Information on MS research quickly hits the media. However, the results of medical research are often overstated— whether by those who did the research, or by those who are reporting it. Tales of sensational improvements help to generate funding, just as they boost TV ratings and newspaper sales. If it sounds too good to be true, it probably is.

At the present time, the most pressing needs in MS research are to discover the exact cause of the disease and to find treatments that work well to stop it, particularly in the case of progressive MS.

Safe MS Drugs

Successfully licensing a drug to treat MS is equivalent to running an obstacle course. A new drug must overcome many hurdles before it can be made generally available.

First, in what is called the preclinical phase, the drug must prove effective and safe in animals: it must suppress an MS-like illness in animals, and not be toxic.

Then, in phase I trials, researchers give the drug to healthy volunteers or to people with MS, to assess its safety and side effects and to get some idea of how well different doses are tolerated. Trials at this stage generally involve a small number of people who are treated for a relatively short time, so the information gained on toxicity is relatively scant.

In phase II trials, a larger group of people in a single center are treated, usually along with a control group receiving a placebo. Phase II trials provide further insight into the safety and side effects of the drug. They also indicate how effective the new treatment probably is. Getting an idea of the effectiveness is crucial because it determines the number of people required for a larger study to prove this effectiveness. What every drug-trial researcher dreads is running a study on a drug that actually works, and having the benefits not show up because the sample of patients was too small. On the other hand, the larger the study, the higher the costs and/or the longer it will have to be run.

In phase III trials, a very large number of people with MS are recruited from different centers—hence the term—"multicenter trial." Typically, hundreds of people are required. They are divided into treatment groups: one group usually receives a low dose of the new medication; one group, a higher dose; and one group, a placebo.

A new drug must succeed in each phase. If it does not work in animals, researchers discard it. If it proves unsafe, researchers discard it. If it does not appear effective in the small, single-center phase II trial, researchers discard it. If it passes phase II but fails the multicenter phase III trial, researchers discard it.

Each phase is more costly than the previous one, and phase III trials are extremely expensive. As well, preclinical, phase I and phase II studies may take a year or more to complete. Phase III trials require several years and millions of dollars.

If, at the end of all this, the drug appears to work and to be safe, the pharmaceutical company that owns the rights to it applies to a regulatory agency—the Food and Drug Administration in the United States, or the Therapeutic Products Program in Canada—for approval to market the drug. Obtaining this regulatory approval can be difficult and time-consuming. In an effort to avoid delays of months or years, these agencies now "fast-track" medications for certain diseases, including MS. Nonetheless, the process still takes a great deal of time.

Once regulatory approval is granted, the pharmaceutical company can market the drug, subject to state and/or provincial prescribing laws and policies. These policies are important because the insurance companies that help pay for the medications typically fall in line with the policies of state or provincial governments. At this point, you can finally get the drug, by prescription, at your local pharmacy.

It is a long, long way from an idea in a scientist's mind to a drug on a pharmacy shelf. The vast majority of ideas don't make it to market. On the other hand, without this careful scientific process, there would be no protection against charlatans selling unproven or even unsafe treatments to people who have enough problems with their MS as it is.

SEVEN

Social Aspects of MS

Different people handle MS differently. Some ignore it and act as if it doesn't exist. Others pay it heed only during attacks; between attacks they try to forget about it. Still others become preoccupied with it, sometimes to the point of obsession. How you deal with MS will depend on your temperament as well as the nature and severity of your symptoms. Economic factors may also affect the way you cope. Symptoms, for example, may become more intense when you are anxious and under pressure.

There is no single "best way" to deal with MS. Whatever works for you and your loved ones is best. But a number of practical issues come up that apply to most, if not all, people with this condition. Here are some thoughts on how to handle them.

Family Life

A potentially disabling disease such as multiple sclerosis obviously has a major impact on family life. Most people with MS come down with it when they are young, just heading toward marriage and starting a family, or in the early stages of family life. MS has the potential to diminish your self-esteem, as you lose the sense of being a healthy person and begin to see yourself as an ill person who has to work at regaining good health and the positive self-image that goes with it.

The person with MS isn't the only one who suffers. Any partner and children also end up paying a price. The partner often sees the person with MS as needier and less capable than the person he or she committed to. This can make the MS sufferer less attractive in general. Many partners send the message: "This is not what I thought I was getting into when I entered this relationship." On the other hand, some partners do remember the principle of "for better or worse, in sickness and in health." Feelings of frustration, even anger, are understandable, particularly if the affected person's needs become greater and his or her ability to contribute to the relationship, emotionally and financially, worsens over time.

Studies have shown that single men with MS are less likely to marry than men without MS, presumably because they are less able to provide economically and emotionally in the ways that make men attractive to women. Some (but not all) studies have suggested that married people with MS have a relatively high divorce rate. Because the demands on a partner become greater as time goes by, a continued willingness to be flexible and helpful is essential.

Children of someone who has MS also have difficulties. On the one hand, they are sorry that the parent is not well and often fear the parent will become disabled or will die. On the other hand, they are frustrated that the parent is unable to keep up with them the way other kids' parents can. Children may even be ashamed to go out in public with a parent who requires a wheelchair or a cane. Both children and partner feel irritated about the demands of the illness, yet guilty about feeling irritated.

Sadly, no easy solutions exist. The partner needs support from other caregivers (physicians, nurses, counselors, social workers), as well as appreciation from the person with MS. Caregiver support groups can also be very helpful in this regard. It helps for health care professionals to tell the couple that MS has two victims: the person with the disease and his or her partner. Just receiving this acknowledgment aids the partner in coping with his or her burden. The same strategy can assist the children.

If you have little or no physical disability, your family lifestyle may not change at all. But many people with MS report that they have had to curtail some of their activities, choosing ones that are less physically demanding and getting more rest if they are going to stay out late. This may disturb your family, because your disability is now affecting them as well.

Therefore, you may have to make some compromises. Instead of pushing yourself to exhaustion, find activities that are less demanding physically but at the same time fun for the rest of the family. Games such as Monopoly, Scrabble or bridge can provide a good excuse for getting together in the afternoon or evening.

Carla is a lawyer who works full-time in spite of having moderate MS. She paces herself carefully, and only accepts evening invitations on the weekend—and then only if she has time for a nap in the afternoon. She's also prepared to come home early if necessary. "If I'm tired, I just leave early and my husband stays longer," she says. "That way I don't feel like

I'm spoiling the evening." By exercising good judgment and self-discipline, she keeps her life as normal as possible.

Many art galleries, museums and shopping malls are now wheelchair accessible. It may be difficult psychologically to use a wheelchair that first time, but it will conserve your energy and allow you to participate more fully and for much longer in family outings.

Pregnancy

Women with multiple sclerosis have no special difficulty becoming pregnant. Does pregnancy have any effect on MS? Yes. During pregnancy—especially in the last three months— MS tends to go into remission. Women notice that their symptoms recede somewhat. As well, flare-ups are relatively uncommon. After the birth of the baby, however—particularly in the first few months—the likelihood of a relapse *increases*. As any mother knows, that first year is filled with physical and emotional stresses, including sleep deprivation, anxiety and hormonal changes. Which of these factors increase the risk of a relapse, we don't yet know.

MS does not affect your ability to give birth. Epidural anesthesia is safe for women with the disease. So is breastfeeding.

Perhaps an important question is, does raising children worsen your MS? No. Several decades ago physicians advised women with MS not to have children, believing that doing so would worsen the disease. We now know this is false.

Still, having a smaller family (one or two children) rather than a larger one is prudent, for purely practical reasons. People with MS have less energy and less earning power, on average. Having a smaller family minimizes the fatigue and financial stress that inevitably accompany parenting. Having children also means you'll be exposed to all the viruses they get—not necessarily a good thing if you have MS. But the final decision, of course, rests with the couple.

Contraception

There are no forms of contraception that affect MS. Oral contraceptives, an intrauterine device (IUD) and sterilization are all used by women with MS without any particular complications. Likewise, the estrogen used in hormone replacement therapy, after menopause, has no known effect on the way MS evolves.

Employment

Without question, MS can negatively affect your employability. Given neurological symptoms such as weakness, numbness, impaired vision and loss of balance, together with fatigue, difficulty in concentrating and memory loss, it's not surprising that employment is often one of the first areas of life to be affected.

The effect is gradual at first. People with MS often notice a lack of energy at work. They may forget things more than they used to. They may be less able to put up with stress, and their concentration may seem to be impaired. They may also feel depressed and burst into tears at times; at other times their emotions are inappropriate. One person, for example, kept breaking into a smile whenever anything was said, even if it was serious or negative, because MS can affect the judgment and emotional centers in the brain. Because the rate of onset of these symptoms of MS is extremely variable—as are all other aspects of the disease—people may be able to continue working for years. Some develop these symptoms almost right away, some many years later and some never develop them at all. Some people become rapidly disabled and their employment difficulties become insurmountable almost as soon as the condition appears, while others never have to give up their jobs because of their MS.

People with physical jobs that require a lot of walking, standing and lifting find MS particularly disabling. It can also be especially disabling for people whose jobs require sustained intellectual effort. On the other hand, sedentary jobs that are more or less routine may be performed for years, if not indefinitely, provided fatigue and impaired concentration are not too severe.

Over the years, researchers have done numerous surveys of employment levels in people with MS. One study found that after 25 years of the disease only a third of the people continued to work. The lower the disability level, the more likely a person was to be employed. A survey of MS patients across Canada, published in 1998, found that 37 percent of those with mild disability were employed in full-time work, compared with 28 percent of those with moderate disability and 4 percent of those with severe disability. Twenty-one percent of those with mild disability did part-time work, as did 10 percent of those with moderate disability and 6 percent of those with severe disability. But many people with MS are homemakers— itself a full-time job—so these statistics are misleading. Perhaps a better way of expressing the difficulty in working is to talk about the unemployment rate of those with MS. According to the same survey, those with mild disability have an unemployment rate of 29 percent; those with moderate disability, 44 percent; and those with severe disability, 77 percent. In the mild group, 37 percent reported a change in employment due to MS, compared with 62 percent in the moderate-disability group and 82 percent in the severe-disability group.

When Should You Tell Your Employer?

People often ask their physicians when they should tell their employers that they have MS. The answer isn't simple, particularly in the early stages of MS. If employers know about the disease, they may be more understanding about medical appointments and generally pick up the slack for the unwell person. But frequently this is not what happens. When disability is minimal—when people have "invisible MS"—they sometimes have to deal with outright hostility from fellow workers and bosses, who resent their frequent absences from work. Sometimes there are complaints about "special treatment."

If you *don't* tell your employer you have MS, you can at least be sure that you won't suffer the subtle discrimination directed at those perceived as less than fit. For example, it might be a career-limiting move for an ambitious junior worker to tell the boss that he or she has MS. Unfortunately, in some instances employers lay off workers for untrue reasons, when the real reason is probably their MS.

When MS is in its early stages, tell people you have the disease on a "need to know" basis, taking into account circumstances and atmosphere. Tell them casually, pointing out that the condition is mild and may well stay that way. It's not wise to spread the news indiscriminately in the early stages; the negatives outweigh the positives.

If the condition becomes "visible," again tell only the people who need to know. By this time supervisors should certainly be informed, so that you can enlist their cooperation and adapt your job so you can continue working.

Look into the benefits plan at your workplace. What are the sick benefits? What are the particulars of the drug plan? Is there coverage for long-term disability? A long-term disability plan is potentially of the greatest financial importance. Don't lightly quit a job that has a long-term disability plan; your next job may not have one. Even if it has, you may be excluded because you had MS prior to being hired. Long-term disability plans vary from company to company. The plans at many large companies pay for a substantial proportion of your regular income up to age 65. Considering that many people with MS are in their thirties or forties, this can be immensely beneficial and can remove a great deal of anxiety about their financial future.

How Can You Enhance Your Employability?
If you can work flexible hours rather than eight straight hours, you're in a better position to continue at a job. Being able to work from home is also an asset. Many people with MS say they cannot work a full day but can work two, three or four hours. If your employer allows part-time work and the insurance company picks up compensation for the remaining part of the day, you'll be able to stay in the workforce much longer. The watchword is *flexibility*. Certain jobs are inflexible by nature, though, or too physical, and people with MS will not be able to continue at them for long. Sometimes these people can be transferred to more flexible, less demanding jobs. In other instances, they will have to quit work and, if they meet the criteria, receive disability insurance from either the government or a private insurance company.

When Should You Go on Sick Leave?
Deciding when to go on sick leave is difficult. It will depend, of course, on how severe the disease is, what the work rules are for sick leave and disability and the general atmosphere of

the workplace. Usually, people with MS are far better off working than not working. Work provides structure in your life. It motivates you and gives you a sense of self-worth. On the other hand, you should not continue when the work causes unbearable physical or emotional stress. Certainly it is far better to collect sick benefits than to be unfairly laid off based on the false perception that you are lazy or are taking excessive time off. Here, disclosing your condition to your employer can be crucial.

Although it varies from jurisdiction to jurisdiction, a social "safety net" generally exists to help everyone with MS one way or another. Look into possible sources of income: sick benefits, disability benefits or pensions, unemployment insurance and welfare. A human resources officer and/or social worker will provide invaluable assistance.

Insurance

Life Insurance

Although people with MS have a potentially disabling disease, their average lifespan decreases by no more than 10 to 15 percent. So it's unreasonable to refuse them life insurance. Premiums, however, may be slightly higher. Certainly the disease is not high-risk in the vast majority of cases. If you have difficulty obtaining life insurance, ask your doctor for help.

Disability Insurance

The fact is that insurance companies are in business to make money. Because people with MS have a high probability of becoming disabled and unable to work, it's almost impossible to get disability insurance with an affordable premium after MS is diagnosed. The key is to have disability insurance before getting sick. That's the only time it's affordable and/or obtainable.

Drug Coverage

Many employment benefit packages include drug coverage. Given the high cost of new disease-modifying therapies in MS, this is a substantial benefit. State or provincial drug plans assist people who do not have insurance, although the rules vary from jurisdiction to jurisdiction.

Car Insurance

Statistically, people with MS are no more dangerous as drivers than anyone else. In fact, they may be safer than average because they tend to drive especially carefully. There is no reason for them not to get automobile insurance, and usually it's not a problem. If your disability is severe enough to interfere with your coordination, or if your arms and legs are weak, it may be necessary to modify your car. For example, if you

---

What every person with MS needs

Everyone with MS needs a family physician who is kind, patient and at least reasonably well informed about MS. He or she should understand that sometimes you may require medical therapy, and other times simply advice. You can't overestimate how much a good family physician can assist in managing MS. If you don't feel comfortable with your physician, find another one. You'll likely have to visit him or her frequently and you'll do better with someone who's on your side.

Everyone with MS also needs a neurologist. He or she will provide as much help as possible, from specific advice to treatment with various drugs. Just knowing what to do is helpful. Treatment for symptoms, and even the underlying disease itself, is available, and researchers are discovering new treatments. If you feel your needs are not being met by your neurologist, find another one.

have weak legs but normal arms you can install hand controls for the gas and brake pedals. When in doubt, it's best to retest your driving skills.

Physiotherapy, Occupational Therapy and Rehabilitation

Many people with MS will see a physiotherapist or an occupational therapist during the course of their disease, particularly after a relapse. Physiotherapists provide exercise programs as well as techniques for maximizing recovery from such problems as weakness and incoordination. They also help you learn to use a cane, walker or wheelchair. Occupational therapists counsel you on how best to function within the confines of your neurological disability. Typically, an occupational therapist will advise you on how to manage fatigue, or how to modify your home or workplace so that you can work around your disability.

Physiotherapists and occupational therapists are both rehabilitation therapists. Rehabilitation aims to attain the best possible neurological function, given the neurological deficit. Rehabilitation therapies (such as exercise programs) are not magic. Some people believe that if they get enough physiotherapy or occupational therapy their neurological deficit will disappear, or significantly dissipate. Unfortunately, this is not often the case. Rehabilitation therapies provide support and direction during the recovery process, so that you can make the most of yourself and your situation. They can improve your self-esteem, your physical fitness and the overall quality of your life.

Given the complex nature of MS, you're wisest to see a physiotherapist or occupational therapist who is familiar with the condition.

Planning for the Future

It's only prudent to plan a home you can live in or a job you can do if you become disabled. That doesn't mean disability is inevitable; it just means that, if you do become disabled, the adjustment will be less upsetting. One woman explains: "At the time of my diagnosis, I was a newlywed. We immediately decided to limit our family to two children instead of three. Although I had no disability, we made up our minds to buy a bungalow rather than a two-story home, and to be more careful financially than we might otherwise have been. It's been years since then and I still have no major disability, but I'm glad we took those precautions."

One of the more difficult problems for a couple is a change in their roles. Partners should discuss such possibilities for the future. Sometimes, a two-income family has to learn to cope on one income. Or someone who has worked at home may have to find an outside job, as well as take on even more responsibility for running the home and caring for the children, if a partner becomes disabled. It's important for the affected partner to offer as much moral support as possible. This eases the burden and maintains cooperation.

Single people diagnosed with MS will want to consider job and marriage plans. Are employment plans realistic? A less demanding job would be more suitable and may have to be planned for. Should you get married? How many children should you have?

George learned that he had MS when he was in his early twenties. Although it was mild, he resolved never to marry, for fear that he'd become a burden on his wife and be unable to support his children. Ten years later, though, his MS remained mild, and he had been promoted several times in his job at the bank. He decided that perhaps his decision had been premature and even pessimistic.

Today George is married and the father of two. He's doing well at work and at home. He's not unaffected by his disease—he has cut down on his workload, and has passed up several opportunities to climb the corporate ladder—but this just gives him more time to enjoy his family.

Professional career counseling firms exist in larger cities. State or provincial vocational rehabilitation departments and manpower centers offer job retraining. The counselor should be helpful in making you aware of options for the future. An MS society support group will put you in touch with people dealing with similar problems.

Travel

Many people with MS have no trouble traveling. If your disability is mild, you need only be prudent in your choice of itineraries, so that you don't wear yourself out. Mountain-climbing may be too much—but then again, perhaps not! If you use a wheelchair, or use a walking aid such as a cane, plan your trip carefully to be sure you'll be able to access all the facilities (bathroom, dining-room, etc.) you'll need.

Be sure medical aid will be readily available if you need it, and tell your physician about your travel plans. He or she can supply you with medication in advance for symptoms you may possibly develop: antibiotics for urinary infections, prednisone for relapses, and so on.

Discuss your problems frankly with staff at travel agencies, hotels, airlines and other service industries, and give them a chance to solve them. Remember that you're not the only traveler with disabilities. As baby-boomers retire and develop health complications, they represent a lucrative market for the travel industry.

Consider Bob's case. Bob had always wanted to go around the world, but after several major attacks of MS he felt his dreams were hopeless. However, after meticulous planning he and his wife were able to take a round-the-world cruise. When Bob was tired, he simply rested in their cabin. At ports of call he had the option of going on an excursion with his wife, or staying aboard. If he stayed on the ship, he could rely on his wife to take pictures, buy souvenirs and fill him in on what he'd missed. At the same time, he felt good knowing that he wasn't limiting the trip for her. The cruise was a great success.

Living with Uncertainty

All of us, healthy or not, live with a degree of uncertainty about the future. Unfortunately, MS attacks at an age when people still feel they have a right to decades of life without disability or disease. Adjusting to the new reality is difficult, and requires lots of patience from the affected person as well as from loved ones and caregivers. It's not an easy task, but many thousands of people with MS have accomplished it.

Planning sensibly for the future means having a will, to avoid legal complications and expenses. A "living will" is also a good idea; if you become unable to make decisions about your life and medical treatment, this document will spell out your preferences. In fact, all of us—not just those with MS—should have these documents prepared, just in case.

Quality of Life

"Quality of life" includes physical function, absence of pain, general health, vitality, social function, emotional and mental health. It's possible to have a good quality of life despite having MS. Unfortunately, given the effects of the disease on mental and physical function, this doesn't happen as often as it should. As disability increases, quality of life—at least in the area of physical abilities—usually deteriorates. On the other hand, the emotional aspects of quality of life often stabilize as you adjust to the fact of having the disease.

To maintain an acceptable quality of life, it's important to obtain all available treatment for your symptoms, and for the condition itself, without letting your MS become the sole focus of your life. You can still take part in almost all the activities that other people enjoy, provided that you have the physical ability, and the common sense to do all things in moderation. It's also crucial to maintain a positive attitude toward life, and to build up a network of social support including loved ones, friends and professional caregivers. Also remember that as you adjust to your condition, accepting but not surrendering, your emotional state will improve.

Remember—it *is* possible to have MS and still lead a full and emotionally rewarding life.

Multiple Sclerosis Societies

Most countries throughout North America and Europe have their own multiple sclerosis societies, such as the National Multiple Sclerosis Society in the United States, and the Multiple Sclerosis Society of Canada. These societies typically raise money for research into the cause and treatment of MS, and for services for people with MS and their families. They provide information and counseling, and host educational programs and workshops. They may pay for some things required by people with MS, such as rehabilitation therapy or walking aids, although they do not as a rule cover the costs of physician or hospital services, or drugs. Depending on the jurisdiction, the society may help support specialized MS clinics.

An increasingly important role of MS societies is to lobby governments on behalf of people with MS—to obtain funding for new medications, for example, or to strengthen the laws relating to the rights and needs of the disabled.

MS societies usually have many local branches. They are an excellent source of information about the disease and how to cope with it, and if they can't solve a problem themselves they may be able to direct you to someone who can.

The MS society is there to support you. To contact your local society, or other helpful organizations, see Further Resources, at the end of this book.

EIGHT

A Final Word

In this book I have tried to describe what multiple sclerosis is, how it can affect you, how it can be diagnosed and, most important, how it can be managed. "Adjustment but not surrender" should be the motto of everyone with this condition. Although MS is a serious and sometimes disabling illness, there is much to be optimistic about as we look to the future. Never before in the history of MS have we been so close to finding the cause and developing truly effective treatments. There has been an explosion of research into the disease, particularly clinical trials of new medications, over the past 15 years. There are now five disease-modifying medications available, with many others in earlier stages of clinical trial evaluation. I firmly believe that in the not too distant future we will discover exactly how this condition develops, and how it can be prevented or cured.

Even today we can deal with the symptoms and underlying disease much better than in the recent past. We also have a much better understanding of the psychological and social impact of the disease, and how to manage those aspects of it. Multiple sclerosis societies exist in all the developed nations, and those in the United States and Canada are particularly effective at raising money for research, providing a wide variety of patient services and lobbying the government on behalf of those with MS.

In summary, a great deal has been accomplished. Although much remains to be done, people with MS can look forward to a future that is much less forbidding than was recently the case. Consider the stories of three people with MS.

Mona was married, with two children aged three and five. She had frequent attacks, with arm and leg weakness and loss of vision in the first few years of her disease. She was naturally very anxious and depressed at the beginning of her illness. About 10 years after the onset of the disease, she entered into the slow progressive phase, and she is now in a wheelchair. Nonetheless, she remains active as a volunteer in the MS society. She gets lots of rest when necessary. She has adjusted to her disability and has no hesitation in declaring that her life is very worthwhile despite the challenges she faces. Her husband and her two teenagers are very supportive, and a source of great happiness.

Robert, on the other hand, has had attacks with symptoms roughly once a year, and they have been moderate in severity. He walks with a slight limp and will sometimes use a cane. However, he remains active in his desk job at the data entry center of a large corporation. He and his wife have a son and daughter, and he is fully active in the community. He is considering going on one of the new disease-modifying therapies that have become available in the last little while. He is determined to remain as active as ever, and not to miss events like his son's soccer practice or his daughter's ballet recital.

Mary has been even more fortunate. All of her attacks have been very mild, involving minor numbness in her arms and legs or partial loss of vision. After each attack, she has had virtually a complete recovery. She has no visible disability, and has mentioned her diagnosis only to her husband and family members. She is the mother of two children and works part-time at the library. She does find it necessary to pace her activity carefully and get extra rest, but she has adjusted completely to her illness and does not think about it frequently. From her point of view, her disease is "invisible," and she fully intends to keep it that way. "The less thought I give my MS, the better," she says.

The challenges faced by those with MS can be great. However, the ability of the human spirit to overcome and manage these challenges is even greater. It's a constant source of inspiration for all of us who deal with people who are coping with this condition.

Some Drugs for Symptomatic Treatment of MS

Generic name	Some brand names	Action
Bladder Problems		
Clonidine	Catapres	urinary antispasmodic
Desmopressin	DDAVP	urinary suppressant
Flavoxate	Urispas	urinary antispasmodic
Imipramine	Tofranil	urinary antispasmodic
Oxybutynin	Ditropan	urinary antispasmodic
Propantheline	Pro-Banthine	anticholinergic
Terazosin	Hytrin	urinary antispasmodic
Tolterodine	Detrol	urinary antispasmodic
Depression		
Amitriptyline	Elavil†, Enovil*	tricyclic antidepressant
Citalopram	Celexa	SSRI
Fluoxetine	Prozac	SSRI
Imipramine	Tofranil	antidepressant
Nortriptyline	Aventyl, Pamelor*	tricyclic antidepressant
Paroxetine	Paxil	SSRI
Sertraline	Zoloft	SSRI
Fatigue		
Amantadine	Symmetrel	CNS stimulant
Methylphenidate	Ritalin	CNS stimulant
Modafinil	Alertec	CNS stimulant
Impotence		
Alprostadil	Caverject, Muse	prostaglandin
Papaverine	Pravatine	vasodilator
Sildenafil	Viagra	diesterase inhibitor
Pain		
Amitriptyline	Elavil†, Etrafon	tricyclic antidepressant
Carbamazepine	Tegretol	anticonvulsant
Cyclobenzaprine	Flexeril	muscle relaxant
Gabapentin	Neurontin	anticonvulsant
Methocarbamol	Robaxin	muscle relaxant
Phenytoin	Dilantin	anticonvulsant
Spasticity		
Baclofen	Baclofen, Lioresal	muscle relaxant
Dantrolene	Dantrium	muscle relaxant
Diazepam	Valium	muscle relaxant
Lorazepam	Ativan	muscle relaxant
Tizanidine	Zanaflex	alpha blocker

†Available in Canada only
*Available in U.S. only
SSRI = selective serotonin re-uptake inhibitor
CNS = central nervous system

continued on next page

Tremor		
Acetazolamide	Diamox	carbonic anhydrase inhibitor
Isoniazid	Isoniazid	antibiotic
Primidone	Mysoline	anticonvulsant
Propranolol	Inderal	beta blocker
Vertigo		
Dimenhydrinate	Gravol	antiemetic
Ondansetron	Zofran	antiemetic
Prochlorperazine	Compazine*, Stemetil	antiemetic
Disease-modifying Drugs		
Interferon beta 1a	Avonex, Rebif	
Interferon beta 1b	Betaseron	
Glatiramer acetate	Copaxone	
Mitoxantrone	Novantrone	

† Available in Canada only
*Available in U.S. only

Glossary

Antiemetic: a drug that reduces nausea.

Attack: *See* **Relapse.**

Autoimmune disease: a disease in which the body's immune system mistakenly attacks the body's own tissues. MS is an autoimmune disease.

Axon: a projection from a nerve cell, used to transmit information to other nerve cells.

Brainstem: part of the central nervous system, linking the base of the brain to the spinal cord.

Catheter: a flexible tube inserted into the bladder to drain away excess urine.

Central nervous system: the brain, spinal cord and optic (eye) nerves; connected to the nerves of the peripheral nervous system, which extend throughout the body.

Cerebellum: part of brain behind the brainstem, controlling balance and coordination.

CNS: *See* **Central nervous system.**

Computerized axial tomography (CT scan): an X-ray technique that assembles multiple images into an image of the brain or other area of the body.

CT scan: *See* **Computerized axial tomography.**

Demyelination: destruction of the nerve cells' protective myelin.

Evoked potentials tests: tests to see how quickly and completely specific nerve signals (visual, auditory, etc.) reach the brain. Signals are usually transmitted more slowly in someone with MS.

Flare-up: *See* **Relapse.**

Glatiramer acetate: a small protein fragment similar to a protein in myelin. Injections of glatiramer acetate seem to help stabilize MS, at least in the relapsing-remitting phase.

Immune system: a complex system that defends the body against viruses and other invaders. Sometimes the system malfunctions; *see* **Autoimmune disease.**

Immunoglobulin: a protein produced by cells that are overactive in MS. A high level of immunoglobulins in spinal fluid may indicate MS.

Interferons: immune-system proteins. Injections of some interferons seem to help stabilize MS, at least in the relapsing-remitting phase.

Magnetic resonance imaging (MRI): a sensitive technique that uses a magnetic field to create an image of the brain or spinal cord.

MRI: *See* **Magnetic resonance imaging.**

Myelin: soft, white, fatty protein protecting and insulating a nerve cell.

Myelitis: inflammation of the spinal cord.

Neurology: branch of medicine concerned with the nervous system.

Neuron: nerve cell.

Plaque: scarred area in the central nervous system, where the protective myelin of many axons is damaged or destroyed.

Primary progressive MS: progressive MS that was not preceded by a relapsing-remitting phase of the disease.

Prognostic: indicating the prognosis (anticipated course) of a disease or medical condition.

Progressive MS: a stage in which the disease grows worse without remissions. Usually preceded by a lengthy relapsing-remitting phase.

Relapse: the appearance of a new neurological symptom, or significant worsening of old neurological symptoms, lasting more than 24 hours and occurring without fever or acute illness.

Relapsing-remitting MS: a stage in which symptoms come and go. Sometimes followed by a progressive stage.

Remission: a period when symptoms temporarily diminish or disappear.

Sclerosis: hardening of tissue. In MS, the scar tissue that forms where myelin has been damaged. Also called plaque.

Secondary progressive MS: progressive MS that begins after a relapsing-remitting phase of the disease.

Spasticity: muscle stiffness, often accompanied by painful cramps or spasms.

Spinal cord: bundle of nerves extending down (and protected by) the spine, connecting the brain to the nerves that extend throughout the body.

Synapse: the microscopic space between nerve cells, across which electrochemical impulses are transmitted.

Tremor: shaking; in MS, usually in the limbs, but occasionally in the head or neck.

Vertigo: a dizzying sensation of spinning; sometimes a symptom of MS.

Further Resources

Support Organizations

U.S.A.

National Multiple Sclerosis Society
733 3rd Ave., New York, NY 10017-3288
Toll-free: 1-800-FIGHT MS (212) 986-3240
www.nationalmssociety.org

Consortium of Multiple
  Sclerosis Centers
c/o Gimbel MS Center at
  Holyname Hospital
718 Teaneck Road
Teaneck, NJ 07666
(201) 837-0727
info.mscare.org

Disability Resource Centre
(A directory of products and
  services)
jj Marketing
1205 Savoy Street, Suite 101
San Diego, CA 92107
Toll-free: 1-800-787-8444
  (U.S. only)
(619) 222-8735
www.blvd.com

Equal Employment
  Opportunity Commission
1801 L Street, NW
Washington, DC 20507
Toll-free: 1-800-669-4000
  (U.S. only)
(202) 663-4900
www.eeoc.gov

Office of Special Education and
  Rehabilitative Services
U.S. Department of Education
400 Maryland Avenue, SW
Washington, DC 20202
(202) 205-5465
www.ed.gov/offices/osers

National Council on Disability
1331 F Street NW, Suite 850
Washington, DC 20004
(202) 272-2004
www.ncd.gov

National Family Caregivers
  Association
10400 Connecticut Avenue
Suite 500
Kensington, MD 20895-3944
Toll-free: 1-800-896-3650
(301) 942-6430
www.nfcacares.org

National Rehabilitation
  Information Center
4200 Forbes Boulevard
Suite 202
Lanham, MD 20706
Toll-free: 1-800-227-0216
  (U.S. only)
(301) 346-2742
www.naric.com

Rehabilitation Institute of
  Chicago
345 E. Superior Street
Chicago, IL 60611
Toll-free: 1-800-354-7342
(312) 238-1000
www.rehabchicago.org

Society for Accessible Travel
  and Hospitality
347 Fifth Avenue, Suite 610
New York, NY 10016
(212) 447-7284
Fax: (212) 725-8253
www.sath.org

Travelin' Talk Network
P.O. Box 1796
Wheat Ridge, CO 80034
(303) 232-2979
www.travelintalk.net

Well Spouse Foundation
P.O. Box 30093
Elkins Park, PA 19027
Toll-free: 1-800-838-0879
(212) 644-1241
www.wellspouse.org

Canada

Multiple Sclerosis Society of Canada
250 Bloor Street East, Suite 1000, Toronto, ON M4W 3P9
Toll-free: 1-800-268-7582 (416) 922-6065
www.mssociety.ca

Accessible Transportation
  Directorate
15 Eddy Street
Hull, PQ K1A 0N9
Toll-free: 1-800-883-1813
www.cta-otc.gc.ca

ARCH: A Legal Resource
  Centre for Persons with
  Disabilities
425 Bloor Street E.
Suite 110
Toronto, ON M4W 3R5
416-482-8255
www.arch-online.org

Association for the
  Neurologically Disabled
  of Canada
59 Clement Road
Toronto, ON M9R 1Y5
Toll-free: 1-800-561-1497
  (outside Toronto)
416-244-1992
www.and.ca

Canadian Association of
  Independent Living Centres
1104–170 Laurier Avenue W.
Ottawa, ON K1P 5V5
(613) 563-2581
Fax: (613) 563-3861
www.cailc.ca

Canadian Council on
  Rehabilitation and Work
500 University Avenue, Suite 302
Toronto, ON M5G 1V7
Toll-free: 1-800-664-0925
416-260-3060
www.ccrw.org

Canadian Human Rights
  Commission
Place de Ville, Tower A
344 Slater Street, 8th floor
Canada Building
Ottawa, ON K1A 1E1
(613) 995-1151
www.chrc-ccdp.ca

Canadian Paraplegic Association
1101 Prince of Wales Drive
Ottawa, ON K2C 3W7
(613) 723-1033
www.canparaplegic.org

Office for Disability Issues
Human Resources Development
25 Eddy Street, Suite 100
Hull, PQ K1A 0M5
Toll-free: 1-800-665-9017
www.hrdc-drhc.gc.ca

Books

Benz, Cynthia. *Coping with Multiple Sclerosis.* London, England: Random House, 1993.

Burnfield, Alexander. *Multiple Sclerosis: A Personal Exploration.* New York: Demos Vermande, 1993.

Halper, June, RN, and Nancy J. Holland, RN, eds. *Comprehensive Nursing Care in Multiple Sclerosis.* New York: Demos Vermande, 1996.

Holland, Nancy J., RN, T. Jock Murray, MD and Stephen C. Reingold, PhD. *Multiple Sclerosis: A Guide for the Newly Diagnosed* (2nd edition). New York: Demos Vermande, 2001.

Horner, Bill. *The Last Dance Is Mine.* Montreal: Optimum, 1992.

Kalb, Rosalind C. *Multiple Sclerosis: A Guide for Families.* New York: Demos Vermande, 1997.

——. *Multiple Sclerosis: The Questions You Have, The Answers You Need.* New York: Demos Vermande, 1996.

Kraft, George H., MD, and Marci Catanzaro, RN, PhD. *Living with Multiple Sclerosis: A Wellness Approach.* New York: Demos Vermande, 1996.

Lander, David L. *Fall Down Laughing: How Squiggy Caught Multiple Sclerosis and Didn't Tell Nobody*. New York: J.P. Tarcher, 2000.

Lechtenberg, Richard, MD. *Multiple Sclerosis Fact Book*. Winnipeg: Login, 1995.

Mendelsohn, Steven. *Tax Options and Strategies for People with Disabilities*. New York: Demos Vermande, 1996.

Pollin, Irene, and Susan K. Golant. *Taking Charge: Overcoming the Challenges of Long-term Illness*. Toronto: Random House, 1994.

Rogers, Judith, and Molleen Matsumara. *Mother to Be: A Guide to Pregnancy and Birth for Women with Disabilities*. New York: Demos Vermande, 1991.

Russell, Margot (ed). *When the Road Turns: Inspirational Stories about People with MS*. Deerfield Beach, Florida: Health Communications, 2001.

Schapiro, Randall T., MD. *Symptom Management in Multiple Sclerosis*. New York: Demos Vermande, 1994.

Sibley, William A., MD. *Therapeutic Claims in Multiple Sclerosis*. New York: Demos Vermande, 1996.

Index

*Page numbers in italic
indicate a figure or boxed
text. For drug brands please
see the table of drug names
on pages 135–36.*

acetaminophen 53
acetazolamide 82
acetylsalicylic acid (ASA) 53
ACTH (adrenocorticotropic
  hormone) 43
acupuncture 53, 95-96
adductor spasms 90
adrenocorticotropic
  hormone (ACTH) 43
aerobic exercises 69
age 13-14
AIDS 35
alcohol 87
allergies
  no link with MS *13*
  risk with venom injection
    99-100
alpha blockers *59*
alprostadil 91

alternative therapies
  acupuncture 53, 95-96
  aromatherapy 96
  chiropractic 96
  cold immersion 96
  dietary supplements 97-98
  herbal medicines 98
  homeopathy 98-99
  massage 53, 100
  meditation 53, 100
  pros and cons 93-95
  reflexology 101
  tai chi 101
  venom injection 99-100
  yoga 101
amantadine 51
American Indians 9
amitriptyline
  for depression 64
  for emotional instability 65
  for tingling 53, 89
anaphylaxis 100
anesthesia *45*
ankles, swollen 84-85
antibiotics *60*

antidepressants
  for anxiety 65
  side effects 64, 85
anti-inflammatory drugs 53
antiseizure drugs 82
anxiety 65
aromatherapy 96
ASA (acetylsalicylic acid) 53
Asian people 9
autoimmune diseases
  about 6-7
  in women 9
Avonex *see* interferon beta:
  1a
axons 3-5
azathioprine 111

baclofen
  for pain 52
  for spasticity 73
balance stimulation 80
bathroom tips 48, 83
baths (therapeutic) 67
bedsores 87-88
bee venom 100
benign MS 37
benzodiazepines 74
beta blockers 81-82
Betaseron *see* interferon
  beta: 1b
biofeedback 53, 80
black people 9
bladder problems
  about 26-27

flaccid big bladder 55-56
incoordinated bladder 56
infections 59, 60
management 56-60
spastic small bladder 54-55
blood tests 33
botulin 75
bowel problems 26-27,
  60-62
braces 77
brain
  illustration 2
  parts and functions 1-3
brainstem 2-3
bulk-forming agents 62
buspirone 65

cancer 35
canes 77-78
capsaicin 53
carbamazepine
  for pain 52
  for spasms 74
cars
  accidents 66-67
  insurance 125-26
Carswell, Robert xi
catheterization 57-58, 60
causes of MS
  environmental associations
    11-15
  genetic associations 9-11
  research 15, 112
celiac diet 86-87

central nervous system 1-2
cerebellar tremor 81-83
cerebellum 3
Charcot, Jean-Martin xi-xii
children of parent with MS
  caring for 49, 119-20
  emotions of 117-18
chiropractic 96
chronic fatigue syndrome 35
cladribine 111
climate 11-13
clinically isolated syndrome
  (CIS) 18, 37
clinical trials 113-14
clonidine 59
codeine 53
cognitive neurorehabilitation
  69-70
cold immersion 96
computerized axial
  tomography (CT) scans
  32-33
computerized balance
  stimulation 80
constipation 27, 61-62
contraception 120
coordination loss 24-25,
  79-80
Copaxone *see* glatiramer
  acetate
corpus callosum 2
corticosteroids
  defined 43
  effects 44-46

for relapses 89
how administered 43-44
side effects *43*, 44-45, 85
use in pregnancy 45
cortisone 43
counseling
  about careers 128
  for anxiety 65
  for depression 63-64
  for sexual problems 92
  for stress 67, 68
cramping, *see also* spasticity
  28, 74
Credé maneuver 57
crutches 78
Cruveilhier, Jean xi
CT (computerized axial
  tomography) scans 32-33
cyclobenzaprine 53
cyclophosphamide 111
cystoscopy 58-59
cytokines 5

dantrolene 74
decadron 43
demyelination 3-5, 7
depression
  about 20-21
  causes 63
  management 63-69
desmopressin 59
diagnosis
  difficulty of 29-30
  process 30, 33-34

reaction to 34-35
similar conditions 35-36
tests 31-33
diarrhea 27, 62
diazepam 74
diet *see* foods
dietary supplements 97-98
dimenhydrinate 80
disability
  and family life 117-19
  insurance 124-25
  planning for the future
    127-29
diuretics
  for swollen ankles 85
  for tremors 82
dizziness 23-24, 79-80
double vision 23
dressings 88
drugs, *see also table on
  pages 135-36*
  causing tremors 81
  for bladder problems 57,
    59-60
  for constipation 62
  for depression 64
  for fatigue 50-51
  for memory problems 70
  for progressive MS 103,
    110-11
  for relapses 43-46
  for relapsing-remitting MS
    103-10

for spasticity 73-74, 75
for tremors 81
for vertigo 80
for weakness 76
insurance coverage 125
research 54, 70, 76, 102-3
dysesthesia 52-53
dysphagia 83-84

employment, *see also* workplace
  enhancing employability
    123
  of people with MS 120-21
  sick leave 123-24
  telling your employer
    122-23
enemas 62
environmental associations
  diet 12
  infections 13-15
  latitude 11-13
  migration 15
  socioeconomic status 13
epidural anesthesia 45, 119
European people 9
evening primrose oil 97
evoked potentials tests 31-32
exercise
  for pain relief 53
  for spasticity relief 71-72
  for stress relief 68-69
  for weight control 86

rehabilitation therapies 126
to aid balance 80
yoga and tai chi 101

Faeroe Islands *14*
family
  history of MS 9-11
  living with MS 116-20
  planning for the future
    127-29
fatigue
  about 19-20, *27*
  drug management 50-51
  non-drug management
    46-50
fatty acids 86, 97-98
fiber 61, *62*
fish oil 86, 98
flaccid big bladder 55-56,
  57-58
flavoxate 57, *58*
fluoxetine 51
flu vaccine *41*, *45*
foods
  and swallowing problems
    84
  as factor in MS *12*, 86-87
  dietary supplements 97-98
  healthy diet 87
  high-fiber 61, *62*
  weight gain 85-86
frontal lobes 2-3

gabapentin
  for pain 52
  for spasms 74
  for tingling 89
gender *see* men; women
genetic associations
  family history 9-11
  racial group 9
  sex 9
genetic research *10*, 112
geography 11-13
glatiramer acetate
  (Copaxone) 103, 108-10
grief *63*

heat massage 53
herbal medicines 98
home
  bathroom tips 48, 83
  energy-saving tips 47-48
  kitchen tips 48-49, 83
  occupational therapist's
    role 47, 126
  safety 49-50
homeopathy 98-99
hormone replacement
  therapy 120
hydrocortisone 43

imipramine 57, 58, 60, 64
immobilization 82
immune system
  about 5

research 112-13
immunizations 41, 45
impotence 26-27, 90
incontinence
  bowel 62
  urinary 26, 54-56, 59
incoordinated bladder 56, 58
infant care 49
infections 13-15, 41
injection therapy
  alternative 99-100
  for relapsing-remitting MS
    104
  for spasticity 75
insurance 124-26
intention tremor 82
interferon beta
  1a (Avonex, Rebif) 103,
    107-8, 109
  1b (Betaseron) 104-6, 109
  about 103
  for memory problems 70
intrauterine devices 120
Inuit 9
isoniazid 82

kidney disease 56
kitchen tips 48-49, 83

Laplanders 9
latitude 11-13
Lhermitte's sign 52
life insurance 124
limbic system 3

linoleic acid 97
living wills 129
loperamide 62
lorazepam
  for anxiety 65
  for spasticity 74
lupus erythematosus 35
Lyme disease 35
lymphocytes 5
lymphoma 35

macrophages 5
magnetic resonance imaging
  (MRI) 31
marijuana 54
marriage 117
massage 53, 100
McDonald criteria 34
mechanical aids for spasticity
  75
meditation 53, 100
memory problems 21-22,
  69-70
men
  bladder infections 60
  catheterization 58, 60
  marriage 117
  passing on MS to children
    10-11
  prevalence of MS 9
  prognosis 38
  sexual problems 89, 90-91
methocarbamol 53
methotrexate 111

methylphenidate 51, 70
methylprednisolone 43
migration 15
mitoxantrone 111
modafinil 51
monoclonal antibodies 112
motor vehicle accidents 66-67
MRI (magnetic resonance
   imaging) 31
Muller (pathologist) xi
multiple sclerosis
   defined 7
   discovered x-xi
   prevalence x, 9-10
   process 3-5, 7
   prognosis 36-39
   social aspects 116-31
   types xii, *37*
multiple sclerosis societies
   130-31
muscle stiffness *see* spasticity
music 67
myelin
   about 3-5
   research 112-13

narcotics 53
natalizumab 113
nausea 80
nerve cells (neurons) 3, *4*
nervous system
   functions 1
   how it works 3-5
   parts 1-3

neuralgia 52
neurologists 30, *125*
neurology xi-xii
neurons (nerve cells) 3, *4*
nortriptyline 64
numbness 25-26, 89

occipital lobes 3
occupational therapists 47,
   126
office *see* workplace
ondansetron 80
oral contraceptives 120
orthoses 75, 77
orthotics 75, 77
oxybutynin
   for bladder problems 57,
      58, 60
   for bowel problems 62

pain 22, 52-53
papaverine 91
parietal lobes 3
pemoline 70
penile vacuum device 91
percutaneous rhizotomy 52
peripheral nervous system 1
personal safety devices 50
phenol 75
phenytoin
   for pain 52
   for spasms 74
physician's role *125*
physiological tremor 81

physiotherapists 69, 80, 126
placebo effect 94
polyunsaturated fatty acids 86, 97-98
potassium channel blockers 76, 112
prayer 67
prednisone 43-44
pregnancy
  and interferon beta 106, 108
  and steroid use 45
  effect on MS 119
  epidurals 45, 119
pressure sores 87-88
primary progressive MS
  defined 19, 37
  management 37-38
primidone 82
prochlorperazine 80
progressive MS
  defined xii, 37
  treatment 103, 110-11
propantheline 57, 58
propranolol 81
prosthesis, penile 91
psychological problems 36

quality of life 129-30

racial group 9
range-of-motion exercises 68-69
Rebif *see* interferon beta: 1a
reflexology 101

rehabilitation 126
relapses
  defined 27, 40
  preventing 42
  steroid treatment for 43-46
  types 42
relapsing-remitting MS
  defined xii, 18, 37
  treatment 37-38, 103-10
relaxation techniques
  for spasticity relief 72-73
  for stress relief 67-68
remissions 27
research
  clinical trials 113-14
  genes 10, 112
  into causes 15, 112
  into symptoms 112
  into treatment 54, 70, 76, 102-3, 111-13, 132-33
resting 46-47
rest tremor 81
rhizotomy 52
rural dwellers 13

safety planning 49-50
safflower seed oil 97
sarcoidosis 35
secondary progressive MS
  defined 19-20, 37
  treatment 37-38
seizures 28
selective adhesion molecule inhibitors 112-13

selective serotonin re-uptake
inhibitors (SSRIs) 64
self-catheterization 57-58
self-image 91-92
sex *see* men; women
sexual problems
about 26-27, 89-90
management 90-93
shaking 24-25, 81-83
siblings 10
signs *see* symptoms and signs
sildenafil 90-91
sleep 47
slurred speech 27-28
snake venom 99
socioeconomic status 13,
14-15
spasticity
about 70-71
drug management 73-74, 75
non-drug management
71-73, 75
surgical management 76
spastic small bladder
54-55, 57
speech difficulties 27-28, 83
spinal cord 1, 3
spinal taps 32
spouses 117-18
SSRIs (selective serotonin
re-uptake inhibitors) 64
sterilization 120
steroids *see* corticosteroids
stimulants 51

stress
coping strategies 67
emotional 65-66
physical 66-68
stretching 71-72
stroke 35
sunflower seed oil 97
sunshine 12
support stockings 85
support systems
at work 124
for caregivers 118
health care professionals
118, *125*, 126
importance *67*, 130
MS societies 130-31
surgery
for facial pain 52
for spasticity 76
safety in MS patients *45*
swallowing problems 83-84
swollen ankles 84-85
symptom management
40-101
symptoms and signs 17-28
age at onset 17
bladder problems 26-27,
55-60
bowel problems 26-27,
60-62
brief and unusual 27-28
defined *18*
depression 20-21, 63-69
dizziness 23-24, 79-80

double vision 23
fatigue 19-20, 27, 46-51
fluctuations 41-42
list of *19*
loss of coordination 23-25,
    79-80
memory changes 21-22,
    69-70
numbness 25-26, 89
onset 17-18
pain 22, 52-53
progression of 17-19
relapses 27, 40, 42-46
remissions 27
research into 112
sexual problems 26-27,
    89-93
shaking 24-25, 81-83
tingling 25-26, 89
unsteadiness 23-24, 79-80
visual loss 22-23
weakness 24, 76-79
worsening of 27
systemic lupus erythematosus
    35

tai chi 101
temperature effects 11, 27,
    86
temporal lobes 3
TENS (transcutaneous elec-
    trical nerve stimulation) 53
terazosin 59
tic douloureux 52

tingling 25-26, 89
tizanidine 74
tolterodine 57
tonic spasms 74
tranquilizers
    for anxiety 65
    for spasticity 74
    for tremors 82
    side effects 81
transcutaneous electrical
    nerve stimulation (TENS)
    53
travel 128-29
treatment, *see also specific*
    symptom
    progressive MS 103,
        110-11
    relapsing-remitting MS
        37-38, 103-10
    research *54*, 70, 76, 102-3,
        111-13, 132-33
tremors *see* shaking
tricyclic antidepressants 64
trigeminal neuralgia 52
twins 10

Uhthoff's phenomenon 27,
    66
ultrasound 53
unsteadiness 23-24, 79-80
urban dwellers 13
urinary system
    illustration *55*
    problems 26-27, 54-60

proper functioning 54
urinary tract infections 27,
  59, 60
urodynamic testing 58-59

Van Bieren, Jan x
venom injections 99-100
vertigo 24, 80
vestibular stimulation 79-80
Viagra (sildenafil) 90-91
vibrators 90
viruses 13-15, *41*
visual loss 22-23
vitamin D 12, 97
vomiting 80

walkers 78-79, 83
walking problems 76-77
water pills
  for swollen ankles 85
  for tremors 82
weakness 24, 76-79
weight gain 85-86

weighting therapy 82
wheelchairs 78-79, 119
white people 9
women
  bladder infections 59, 60
  catheterization 58, 60
  marriage 117
  passing on MS to children
    10-11
  pregnancy 45, 106, 108,
    119
  prevalence of MS 9
  prognosis 38
  sexual problems 89, 90
workplace, *see also*
  employment
  energy-saving tips *50*
  occupational therapist's
    role 47, 126
  stress 66

yoga 101